Essential Obstetric Practice

For Trudie, Alexandra and Stephanie

Essential Obstetric Practice

Gerald J. Amiel MB, BS, MRCS, FRCOG

Examiner to the Central Midwives Board

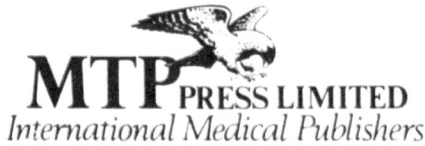

Published, in association with
Hastings Hilton Publishers Limited,
by

MTP PRESS LIMITED
International Medical Publishers

Published, in association with
Hastings Hilton Publishers Limited,
London,

by

MTP Press Limited
International Medical Publishers
Falcon House
Lancaster, England

First published 1981

ISBN-13: 978-0-85200-361-9   e-ISBN-13: 978-94-011-7233-2
DOI: 10.1007/978-94-011-7233-2

Phototypesetting by Swiftpages Ltd., Liverpool

Contents

Introduction

Advances in research, knowledge and clinical practice in all branches of medicine have been rapid over the past decades and the speed is accelerating. Thus, as we enter the 1980s the pressure on specialists is to concentrate on ever-narrowing fields of their science. For the research worker this is desirable, but the practising clinician can have no clearly defined dividing lines. Our patient is a whole individual and every aspect of her makeup, physical and psychological, must always be taken fully into account. This is of vital importance in obstetrics and gynaecology. These two closely inter-woven disciplines are branches of medical science in which emergency situations are not uncommon. Thus every practitioner, doctor, mid-wife and nurse needs understanding of these subjects. Although technology advances rapidly, many basic principles remain the same. The chapters that follow deal with these, and modern trends in clinical management are discussed.

For some decades the author has been in clinical charge of a maternity hospital some 12 miles south of Central London. The hospital is a training school for obstetricians and midwives, and the local population is adequately supplied with a general practitioner service. These circumstances are of some relevance because many views expressed are based on personal experience while others are based on countless books, articles, congresses and discussion with colleagues. To every source of information I express my thanks.

Obstetrics or midwifery (I regard the terms as synonymous) is an art. Above all, it is a gentle art. One of the essential features of the practice of obstetrics is the fact that there can be no hard and fast rules to govern management. Each case is assessed individually and then reassessed at every subsequent examination before deciding upon the nature of the recommendations to be made to the patient. Furthermore, management may differ according to the facilities available in a particular area. Thus, in many parts of the world the obstetrician may rightly be more reluctant to perform caesarean section if it is considered that the patient will not have ready access to skilled medical attention in a properly equipped institution in her next pregnancy. Conversely, although caesarean section as a mode of delivery carries extra risks to both mother and baby, a long labour followed by difficult vaginal delivery has little to commend it either in the United Kingdom or the United States.

Improvement in maternal and perinatal mortality and morbidity is brought about by a variety of factors which include:

(1)   The standards of, and facilities for, antenatal care.

(2)   Screening techniques for mother and fetus which may exclude abnormal conditions or alert the practitioner to potential hazards.

(3)   The early recognition and treatment of complications of pregnancy.

(4)   The management of labour, the place of delivery and the skill of the midwifery team.

(5)   The care of the newborn.

During parturition a baby passes through the bony pelvis and meets some resistance from the soft parts, and especially the muscles of the pelvis floor. A knowledge of basic anatomy is necessary, and the trend of many textbooks to commence with this subject is wise and followed in this volume. The consideration of some topics, however, does not follow a usual routine. Thus, for example, the management of the third stage of labour and postpartum haemorrhage follows immediately the description of the physiology of labour, and diabetes fits naturally into a chapter discussing abnormal constituents in urine. Physiology, histology, endocrinology and bacteriology all have important roles in obstetrics and principles of these subjects are included.

Some of the text follows that of articles published in a series on obstetrics in *Update Journal of Postgraduate General Practice* during 1978. Other parts are based on a series of lectures given to numerous classes of students. It is hoped that readers studying obstetrics will find in this volume a fresh approach to the subject which will enable them more readily to assimilate the material and by so doing improve their knowledge and care of the pregnant woman.

I am grateful to the Editor of *Update* for permission to use some of the material published. Also my thanks to Dr Stephanie A. Amiel for helpful advice, and to my wife whose help in the preparation of the typescript was invaluable.

1

Anatomy

The pelvis

The bony pelvis is, as the Latin derivation of the name denotes, a 'basin' and it is through this bony passage that the baby has to pass in the process of parturition. In the normal course of events the head of the fetus leads, and passes in and out of the pelvis without much difficulty even though there is not too much room to spare. The pelvis contains a few joints and is thus capable of stretching or 'give' when subjected to pressure by the passage of the baby during labour, but the amount of 'give' is very limited. The shape of the pelvis is important and the midwifery practitioner needs a knowledge of some of its measurements and angles to be able to make the correct decision for safe delivery of the infant.

Obstetrics is concerned with the bony pelvis as a whole and not with the individual bones that comprise it. However, a better understanding is achieved if initially the individual bones are considered. The description that follows is that of the *gynaecoid* pelvis which is typically the normal female pelvis and that best adapted for childbirth. Minor variations in shape or size occur in more than 50 per cent of women, but more gross abnormalities will lead to difficulties in labour (*dystocia*) and are discussed in Chapter 18.

The pelvis is formed by the two *innominate* bones which meet anteriorly at the symphysis pubis, and posteriorly articulate with the sacrum (Figure 1). Each innominate bone is formed by three bones:

(1) *The ilium*, the flattened superior portion which has a long curved upper border, the iliac crest. The crest may be felt quite easily through the skin for much of its extent even in adipose patients.

(2) *The ischium*, the lower posterior portion which contains two important prominences:
    (a) the tuberosity, a large knob of bone (on which we sit);
    (b) the ischial spine, a smaller, sharper projection medially which projects to a variable degree into the pelvic cavity.

1

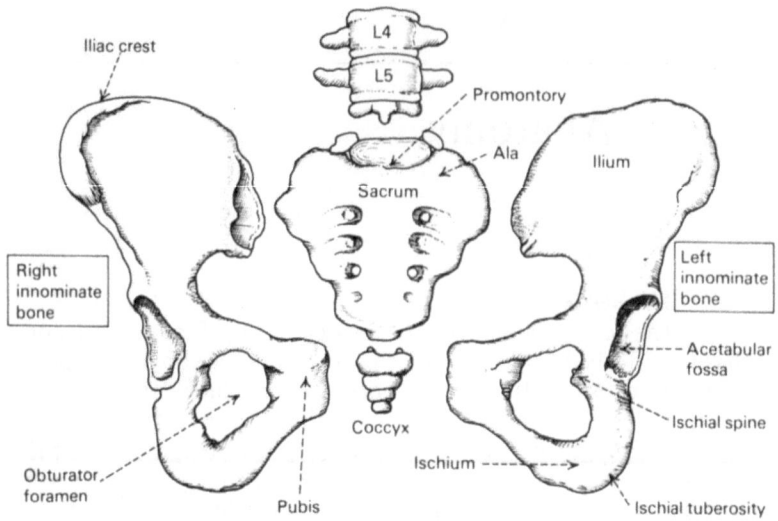

Figure 1   Individual bones of the pelvis

(3)   *The os pubis.* This, the anterior part of the innominate bone meets its fellow in the midline to form a cartilaginous joint, the *symphysis pubis.* Basically each pubic bone consists of a flat plate, with upper and lower projections, the superior and inferior rami.

The three individual bones that comprise the innominate bone unite with each other in the deep socket which receives the head of the femur, that is the *acetabular fossa.* Below and anterior to the acetabulum is the *obturator foramen*, a large oval gap which in life is covered by the thin obturator muscle.

The *sacrum* is a curved and triangular-shaped bone which consists usually of five fused vertebrae (Figure 1). The anterior surface of the gynaecoid sacrum has a shallow concavity, and its shape is important in determining the available space of the pelvic cavity. The superior border of the sacrum (the first sacral vertebra) has a body with an anterior projecting edge, the *sacral promontory* – from which the wings or *alae* pass to the sacroiliac joints. Attached to the inferior border of the sacrum is the *coccyx* which usually consists of four fused vestigial vertebrae, although occasionally the number may be three or five. The *coccyx* is the rudimentary tail bone, and there is a small disc of fibrocartilage at its articulation with the sacrum. The coccyx is pushed backwards in labour, but if there is excessive trauma a patient may be left with a 'painful coccyx' (*coccydynia*).

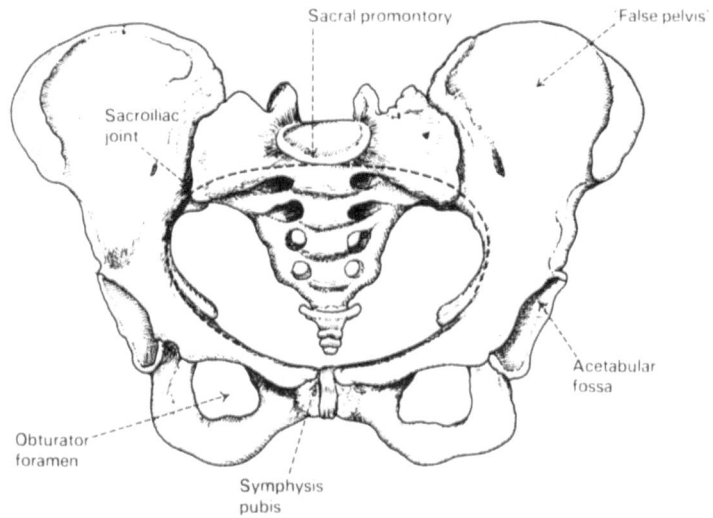

Figure 2   The articulated pelvis

As the articulated pelvis as a whole is important in obstetrics and not the individual bones, it is convenient to divide the pelvis into:

(1) *The false pelvis*, which is the splayed-out upper part of the ilium, and
(2) *The true pelvis*, which comprises the pelvic brim and all below.

The boundaries between these two zones are clearly defined and may be seen in Figure 2 and in the models used in teaching the subject. The measurements of the false pelvis or whether or not a woman has broad hips are irrelevant today. It is the true pelvis that is important, and this is assessed clinically and occasionally by radiology. In every pelvis the zones to consider are:

(1)   The pelvic brim or inlet (entrance to the true pelvis).
(2)   The cavity.
(3)   The outlet.

The borders of the pelvic inlet are shown in Figure 3 and it is of fundamental importance in midwifery to be completely familiar with them. The brim is circular with the sacral promontory projecting into its posterior aspect. It is not 'heart-shaped'. The posterior boundaries

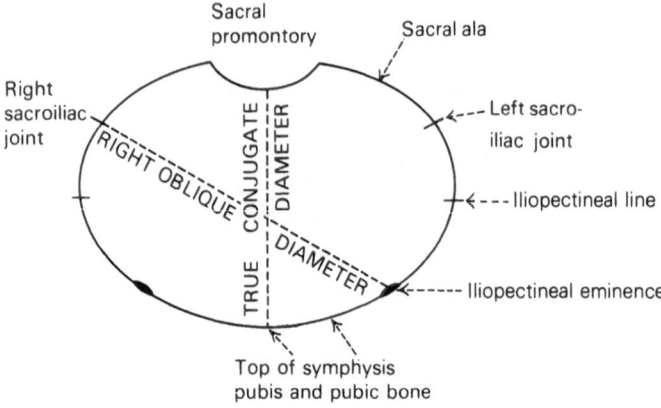

Figure 3   Boundaries of pelvic inlet from above

are the sacral promontory with the sacral alae extending to the sacroiliac joints. Anteriorly, in the midline is the top of the symphysis pubis and pubic bone with its upper arm or superior ramus. The remainder of the brim consists of a well-defined bony ridge in the ilium — the *iliopectineal line* — which extends to a thickened boss called the *iliopectineal eminence*.

The *anteroposterior* diameter of the inlet extends from the middle of the sacral promontory to the top of the symphysis pubis and is the most important single measurement of the pelvis. It is also called the *true conjugate* diameter of the pelvis and on average measures 11 cm. The *oblique* diameters (12 cm) extend from the sacroiliac joint to the opposite iliopectineal eminence and the side is named to accord with the sacroiliac joint from which it extends (in other words, the right oblique diameter is that which passes from the right sacroiliac joint to the left iliopectineal eminence). The *transverse* diameter is the maximum transverse measurement and averages 13 cm. The measurements given are approximations for European women, and there are racial differences in addition to wide individual variation.

The *pelvic cavity* has an irregular shape and is bounded by the pubic bones in front, the inner surfaces of ischium and ilium at the sides and the anterior surface of the sacrum and coccyx posteriorly. The side walls of the gynaecological pelvis do not converge, nor do the ischial spines project excessively into the cavity. As stated earlier, the anterior surface of the sacrum should show a shallow concavity. If it were straight as in the typical male sacrum or, worse still, if it projected forwards with a convexity, the space available in the pelvic cavity would be diminished. A plane through the middle of the cavity should be circular with a diameter of approximately 13 cm.

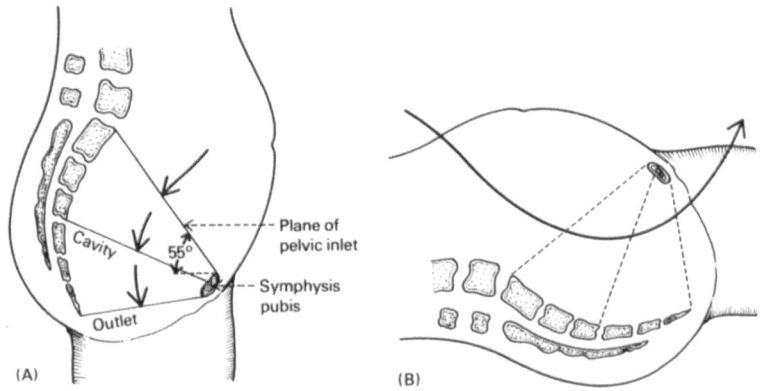

Figure 4   (a) and (b) Pelvic planes

The *pelvic outlet* is a diamond-shaped canal bounded anteriorly by the inferior aspect of the symphysis pubis and the descending rami extending to the ischial tuberosities. The posterior portion of the outlet consists of the sacrotuberous ligaments passing between the ischial tuberosities and the bottom of the sacrum and coccyx. It is the anterior half of the outlet which is of importance in obstetrics and this is the *subpubic arch* extending to the tuberosities. The gynaecoid arch is rounded, the subpubic angle is approximately a right angle, and the interischial diameter between the two tuberosities approximates 12 cm (the transverse diameter of the outlet).

PELVIC INCLINATION

In the erect posture, the plane of the pelvic inlet in European women makes an angle of 50 to 60 degrees with the horizontal. The tilt of the pelvis at various levels is significant because the fetus, placenta and membranes (the so-called 'passengers') follow a curved course during delivery. Figure 4(a) indicates the angles at various levels in the pelvis and the arrow in Figure 4(b) shows the direction taken by the 'passengers' during labour. It can be seen that there is a marked change of direction in the birth canal at the outlet at the pelvic floor level. Knowledge of this is of special importance in the management of the third stage of labour.

CLINICAL EXAMINATION OF THE PELVIS
Internal pelvimetry
The true pelvis is assessed mostly by vaginal examination with two fingers, and is more conveniently performed with the patient in the left

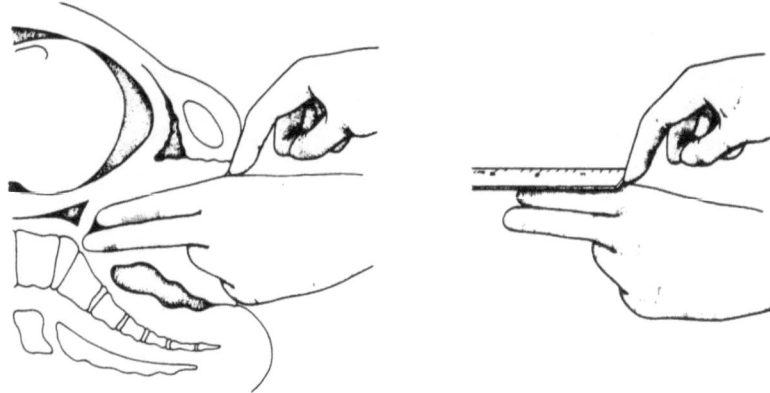

Figure 5   The diagonal conjugate diameter of the pelvis

lateral position. Two fingers of the right hand intravaginally palpate the anterior surface of the sacrum which should have a gentle concave surface. If the pelvis is adequate most doctors are unable to reach the sacral promontory and, in fact, one cannot say this point has been reached unless it is possible to palpate beyond it. If it is identified, the diagonal conjugate may be measured (Figure 5), and is approximately 1 cm more than the true conjugate. The pelvic cavity is further explored by gently sweeping the fingers around in a circular movement; the ischial spines should not be a prominent feature.

External pelvimetry
The pelvic outlet is assessed by pressing the four knuckles between the ischial tuberosities, and the subpubic angle by placing the index finger of each hand along the descending rami of the pubes (Figure 6). The subpubic angle should approximate 90 degrees. Fists differ considerably in size but after a few such examinations most practitioners are able to assess deviations from the average by comparison. Patients should always be informed before estimating the pelvic outlet in this fashion. To insert a fist into the buttocks of a patient suddenly and without prior warning may be psychologically traumatic!

Radiological pelvimetry
In selected cases a lateral pelvimetry X-ray may be taken in the latter days of pregnancy or in early labour. This can be a useful aid to clinical judgement. An inlet view is not requested during pregnancy when exposure to every form of radiation should be kept to a minimum. Such a picture, however, is sometimes taken weeks after

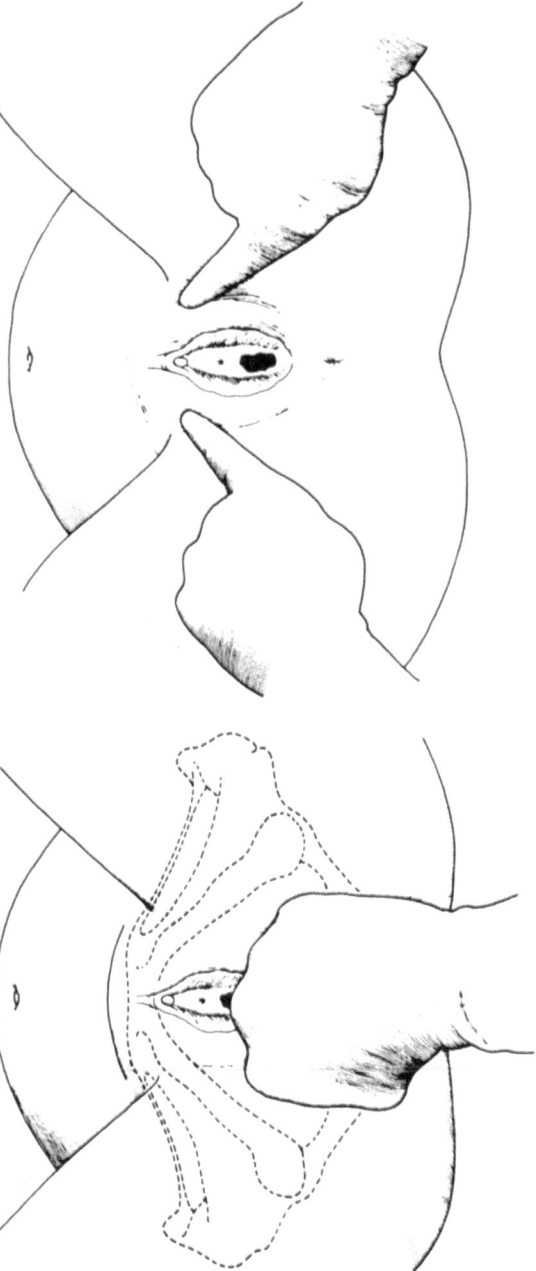

Figure 6   Clinical estimation of the pelvic outlet

labour has ended, to aid judgement of the best mode of delivery in a subsequent pregnancy. The pelvic outlet can be determined clinically and more effectively than with any X-ray picture.

In conclusion it should be noted that in the latter days of pregnancy the baby's head itself is perhaps the most important 'pelvimeter' and if engaged indicates an adequate pelvic inlet and cavity.

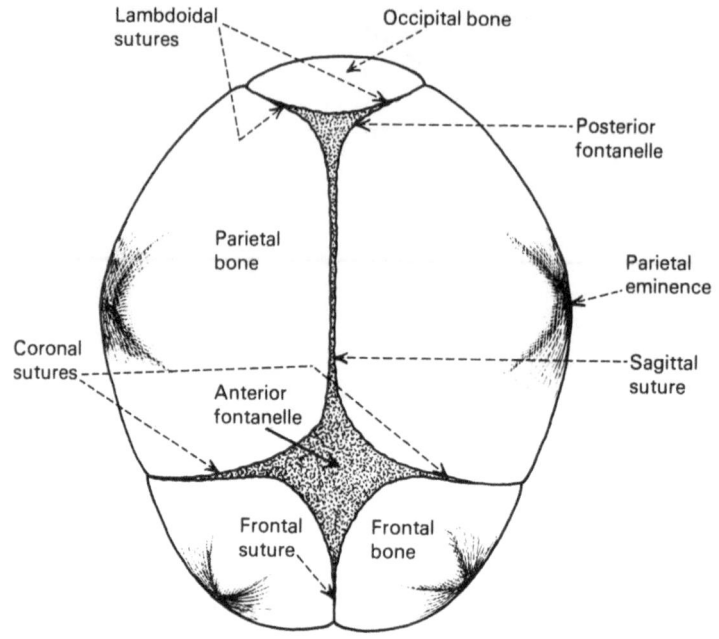

Figure 7   Vault of the fetal skull − landmarks

The fetal skull
If the baby's head can pass in and out of the pelvis, with but few exceptions the rest of the baby will follow without difficulty. Unfortunately for all learning our subject (and sometimes for the patient herself!) the fetal skull is not a sphere and many of its various diameters differ in length. It is thus important to be able to recognize precisely which area of the head is passing through the birth canal, and this is made possible by identifying the 'landmarks' on the vault of the skull when performing a vaginal examination in labour. What then are these landmarks and what is their significance?

The bones of the vault and sides of the skull arise from *membrane* and not from cartilage as do most other bones. Ossification of the membranes commences in early intrauterine life but is incomplete at birth. Hence linear areas of membrane, or *sutures*, persist at birth and these may be identified on vaginal examination. Where three or four sutures meet, a membranous space or *fontanelle* is formed. The bones of the base of the skull, as those of the face, are firmly united at birth and thus incompressible, a feature which enables them to protect vital centres in the brain.

The two largest bones on the crown of the head are the *parietals* each of which posteriorly has a small protuberant area, the *parietal eminence*. Between the parietals in the midline is the *sagittal suture* (Figure 7) which in most labours is the landmark first felt on vaginal examination. Anteriorly, in the region of the forehead are the *frontal bones* separated from each other by the *frontal suture*. The *coronal sutures* lie between parietal and frontal bones. Posteriorly is the *occipital bone* with the two *lambdoidal sutures* between it and the parietals. The prominence on the occiput is the *occipital protuberance* which may be felt readily subcutaneously at the upper end of the median groove at the back of the neck (the nuchal furrow). The large oval aperture in this bone, the *foramen magnum*, is the opening through which brain and spinal cord communicate.

The sides of the vault of the skull are occupied by the *temporal bones* separated from the parietals by temporal sutures. There are fontanelles at the anterior and posterior extremities of these sutures, but they are not as significant in obstetrics as the two described below.

The anterior fontanelle or *bregma* is a large diamond-shaped membranous space where four sutures meet (sagittal, frontal and two coronals). It measures approximately 4 cm anteroposteriorly and 2.5 cm transversely, and it does not close or ossify until the baby is about 18 months old.

The posterior fontanelle or *lambda* is a much smaller triangular space formed by the junction of three sutures (two lambdoidal and the sagittal), and although ossification varies in its timing it is generally completed within 3 months of birth.

Although the fontanelles vary considerably in size, it is wise wherever possible to ensure accuracy in diagnosis by palpating and counting the number of sutures that converge to form the space; if four meet the space is the anterior fontanelle.

The correct identification of these landmarks will show:

(1)   The exact position of the occiput – by considering the disposition of the lines forming the Y-shaped junction of the posterior fontanelle.

(2)   The degree of flexion of the head. If the posterior fontanelle is readily felt on vaginal examination in labour the head is fully flexed, and if the anterior fontanelle is more easily accessible it is poorly flexed (not to be confused with an extended head).

DIAMETERS

Some important diameters of the fetal skull are shown in Figure 8 and will be discussed further when mechanisms of labour are described. A study of a model of the skull with the right index finger inserted into the foramen magnum to represent the fetal spine will help to make the measurements more meaningful than any diagram. With the left hand place the index finger slightly below the occipital protuberance and the thumb on the bregma. This indicates the diameter of engagement in a fully flexed head (the suboccipito-bregmatic 9.5 cm) and also shows the central position of the posterior fontanelle. Slowly deflexing the head with the right thumb observe how the left thumb slips to the frontal bone and the index finger moves to the occipital protuberance, as the anterior fontanelle becomes increasingly central. The suboccipito-frontal (10 cm) and occipito-frontal (11 cm) diameters are those engaging when the head is not fully flexed.

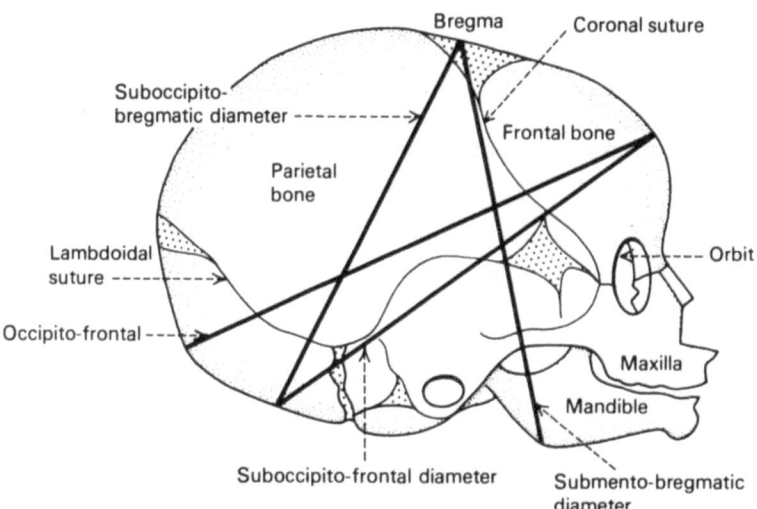

Figure 8   The fetal skull − diameters

REGIONS OF THE SKULL

Four regions are described:

(1) The *vertex*, the area bounded by the anterior and posterior fontanelles and the two parietal eminences.

(2) The *sinciput* or brow, consisting of the frontal bones (from coronal sutures to the orbital ridges).

(3) The *occiput*, which extends from the posterior fontanelle to the foramen magnum.

(4) The *face*, from the root of the nose (glabella) to the junction of chin and neck.

MOULDING

This is a change in the shape of the skull which may occur by pressure on the baby's head during its passage through the birth canal. It is made possible by the presence of the membranous sutures which allow the soft bones to override one another. The parietal bones will usually override the frontal and occipital bones, and the posterior parietal will pass beneath the anterior one due to the greater pressure from the sacral promontory. This phenomenon may enable a tightly fitting head to be delivered spontaneously especially when uterine contractions are strong. There is, however, an increased risk to the fetus of intracranial haemorrhage if moulding is excessive.

At this point it is pertinent to consider two swellings of clinical importance found on the newborn baby's head, caput succedaneum and cephalohaematoma.

CAPUT SUCCEDANEUM

During labour, and usually after the forewaters have ruptured, the ring of the cervix, or less commonly the vagina or vulva, may exert pressure on the presenting part of the scalp and obstruct the venous and lymphatic flow in the area. The resulting congestion causes a boggy ill-defined swelling in and under the scalp due to an effusion of tissue fluids and even blood into the soft tissues. This is the caput succedaneum. The swelling is, as stated, ill-defined, pits on pressure, is present at birth and disappears entirely within 48 hours. It crosses suture lines, and although a normal occurrence the swelling is more marked during prolonged labour.

CEPHALOHAEMATOMA

This swelling is due to haemorrhage which takes place under the periostium of the skull. Although more commonly associated with a traumatic delivery, cephalohaematomata may occur in an apparently easy spontaneous delivery. Swellings are occasionally bilateral and investigations to exclude abnormal bleeding tendencies may be indicated. The swellings will not pit to pressure, do not appear until hours or even a few days after birth, are circumscribed and never cross the suture lines of a bone. They may take many months to absorb and often become hard and calcified before they do so. Vitamin K is often administered and only on rare occasions is the blood aspirated.

The vulva or external genitalia

The external genitalia (Figure 9) are bounded by the outer lips or *labia majora*. These consist of folds of skin with subcutaneous fat, connective tissue, fascia and some involuntary muscle fibres. The fat is continuous with a pad of tissue over the pubis – the *mons veneris* – while posteriorly the labia are joined by a thin fold – the *posterior commissure*. The skin contains hair follicles, sebaceous and sweat glands, and specialized forms of the latter – large, coiled apocrine glands the secretion from which has a characteristic odour. The labia majora contain the ends of the round ligaments of the uterus (see below, page 18), and situated in the posterior third are the *glands of Bar-*

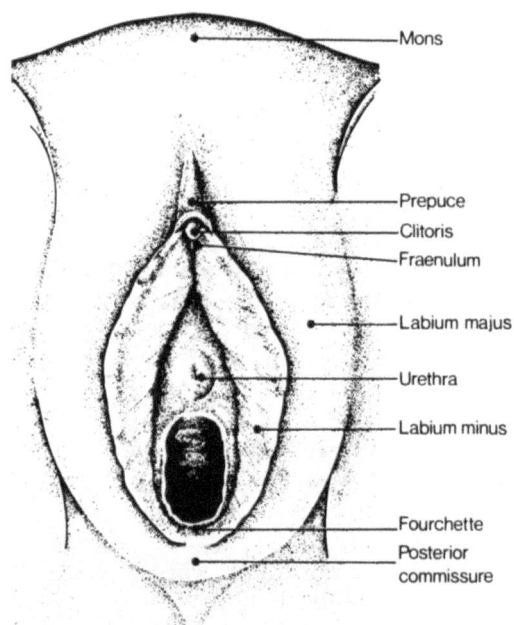

Figure 9 The vulva

tholin, which secrete mucus that plays a small part in lubrication of the lower vagina and vulva. The main duct of each gland opens into the midlateral margin of the vagina and if blocked may lead to a Bartholin cyst which may then become secondarily infected and form an abscess. Bartholin abscess may also be associated with gonorrhoea.

When the labia majora are separated, the *labia minora* are seen. These are double folds of skin with no subcutaneous fat, no hair follicles and few sweat glands. Sebaceous glands, however, are present in abundance. Anteriorly the skin encircles the clitoris, the superior fold being called the *prepuce*, and the inferior fold the *fraenulum* or fraenum. The *clitoris* is composed of muscular erectile tissue, and is the counterpart or homologue of the penis while the labia majora represent the scrotum. Posteriorly the labia minora fuse to form the *fourchette*, a delicate fold which is torn in childbirth.

The *hymen*, a double fold of membrane of squamous epithelium contains fibrous tissue and blood vessels and normally partly occludes the vaginal orifice. If excess fibrous tissue is present the hymen may be *rigid* and cause painful coitus or *dyspareunia*. The latter may well lead to spasm of the muscles around the vagina (*vaginismus*) which in turn increases the pain. A vicious circle is thus set up making normal coitus impossible. The patient may be able to solve this problem herself by digital dilatation of the hymen using lubricant on her fingers, but sometimes hymenectomy under general anaesthesia is necessary. If the hymen is very vascular there may be haemorrhage when it is ruptured and treatment may entail locating and tying off a bleeding point.

Occasionally the hymen may occlude the vagina completely, and the imperforate hymen will not allow menstrual blood to escape (*crypto-menorrhoea*). The vagina is capable of enormous distension and it may take many years of menstruation before a patient realizes that something is amiss.

After vaginal delivery the hymen is destroyed and the tags that remain are known as *carunculae myrtiformes*.

The triangular area bounded by the clitoris, labia minora and vagina is referred to as the *vestibule*. It contains the external urethral orifice or urinary meatus. The *urethra* passes upwards and backwards parallel with the anterior vaginal wall to which it is attached; it is approximately 4 cm long but is lengthened in pregnancy and labour. Small mucous glands open into the urethra and clusters of these are grouped together on each side near its lower end and drain into the *paraurethral ducts* (Skene's ducts). The latter run a tortuous course below the mucosa of the vestibule to open into the lateral margin of the meatus.

The *bladder*, which is capable of great distension, is partially covered with peritoneum (or serous coat, see Figure 10) and has a muscular layer (the detrusor) and inner mucous membrane of transitional epithelium. This is pale pink in colour and thrown into folds (*rugae*) when the bladder is empty. The *trigone* is the smooth triangular area in the mucosa between the orifices of the urethra and the two ureters. The latter run from the pelves of the kidney behind the peritoneum and enter the pelvis near the sacroiliac joints. As they pass downwards and medially to enter the base of the bladder at the trigone, they lie in close proximity with the lateral fornix and supravaginal cervix, a feature of considerable importance to the gynaecological surgeon.

The vagina

The vagina is a fibromuscular tube which passes upwards and backwards from the vulva to the cervix of the uterus. The outer coat forms a sheath of fibrous connective tissue and overlies a middle coat of involuntary or non-striated muscle fibres. There is some differentiation of the latter into outer longitudinal and inner circular fibres but these layers are not clearly defined and much of the musculature consists of oblique crisscrossing fasciculi. A subepithelial layer of elastic connective tissue contains numerous veins and lies beneath the inner mucous membrane. This lining mucosa consists of a stratified squamous epithelium which normally contains no glands whatsoever. The vagina in young adults and especially in pregnancy is, however, generally moist, and the secretion comes from the cervix and corpus uteri and by a process of transudation from the deeper layers. These secretions and those of Bartholin's glands are alkaline in reaction, but the healthy vagina is acid, with a pH value normally between 3.5 and 5.5. This acidity is caused by the presence of *Döderlein's bacilli*, large rod-shaped organisms which react with glycogen liberated from cells shed from the superficial layers of the mucosa to form lactic acid.

It is of interest to note that years ago an international classification of vaginal health was proposed, based upon the acidity and bacterial flora found when a swab was cultured. The healthiest vaginae were acid and contained only Döderlein's bacilli. Second category vaginae were less acid and contained Döderlein's bacilli plus infecting organisms. The least healthy vaginae were alkaline in reaction and cultures grew infecting organisms only.

The anterior and posterior walls of the vagina are normally in contact with each other and each contains a longitudinal ridge (vaginal column). Much more prominent, however, are the numerous transverse folds or *rugae* which extend from the columns. The vagina

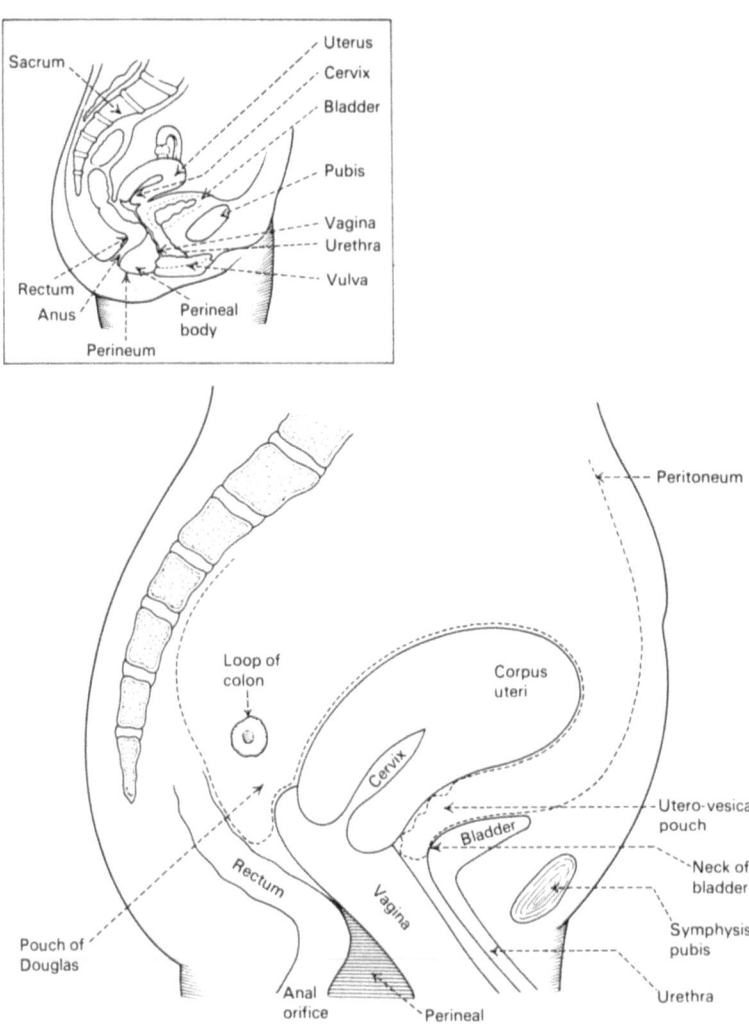

Figure 10   Sagittal view showing relationships of pelvic viscera

grows a little during pregnancy, but the enormous distension it undergoes during the passage of the fetal head in labour is made possible by the unfolding of the rugae so that the membrane becomes a smooth sheet.

The cervix projects into the anterior part of the vaginal vault which is thereby divided into four areas called *fornices*. The posterior fornix is the deepest space and the anterior fornix the most shallow. The ureters passing to the bladder cross the pelvis close to the two lateral fornices.

The relationships or proximities of the vagina are best learnt by studying Figures 10 and 11 and being able to reproduce them with accuracy. In fact the two figures contain many details of the female pelvic anatomy and I consider that simple line diagrams are of most value.

Figure 10 illustrates that the anterior vaginal wall is related to the urethra, neck of bladder and uterovesical pouch of the peritoneum, while the posterior wall, which is much longer (10 cm +), is related in

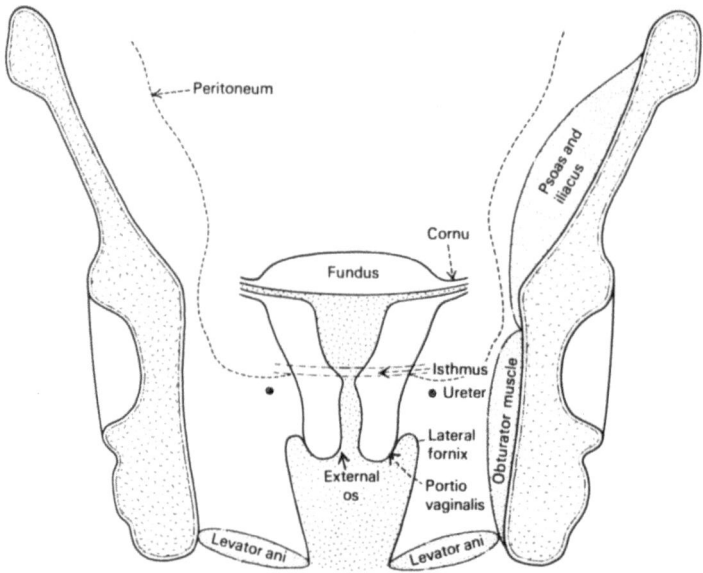

Figure 11   Diagrammatic representation of pelvis to show levels of peritoneum and pelvic floor

its lower third to the perineal body, then is in direct contact with the anterior wall of the rectum, while the upper third is related to the pouch of Douglas. Lateral to the vagina are the pelvic fascia and

levatores ani, while the vaginal orifice is surrounded by a muscle called the bulbo-cavernosus (or bulbo-spongiosus – see page 22).

The uterus
The uterus, a thick-walled muscular organ, is flattened from before
backwards, and the old description comparing its shape to that of a
flattened pear is apt. In the non-pregnant state it measures 7.5 cm in
length, is 5 cm wide and 2.5 cm thick (these measurements were
originally easier to learn – 3 by 2 by 1 inch!). The uterus has but one
function only and that is to receive, embed and nourish the fertilized
ovum. The thick wall which encloses a small triangular-shaped cavity
consists of three layers:

(1)   The outer peritoneal coat – perimetrium.
(2)   The middle muscular coat – myometrium.
(3)   The inner mucosal coat – endometrium.

The arrangement and action of the muscle fibres in late pregnancy
and labour and the marked cyclical changes of the endometrium are of
importance and are considered in some detail below (pages 176 and 27).
  The uterus consists of the body or *corpus*, and the *cervix* which is
the lower third. Between these two areas is a narrow zone, the
isthmus, which has slight differences histologically from both corpus
and cervix, and which with the latter takes part in the formation of the
lower segment in labour. The fallopian tubes enter the corpus uteri at
the *cornua* (singular: cornu) above which is the *fundus* of the uterus.
  The cervix (2.5 cm long) projects through the anterior part of the
vaginal vault so that about two-thirds is supravaginal, the rest being
the portio vaginalis or vaginal part. The inner endocervical canal is
fusiform in shape, that is, wide in the middle and narrow at both ends
(these being the internal and external os). The canal or endocervix is
lined with a mucous membrane of tall epithelial cells containing
branching (racemose) glands which secrete a thick alkaline mucus.

POSITION OF THE UTERUS
The normal position of the uterus is one of *anteversion* which means
the cervix is pointing forwards from the external os, and *anteflexion*
which signifies that the body is bent forwards on the cervix.
  If the cervix pointed backwards the position would be described as
retroverted, and retroflexion would indicate that the corpus uteri was
bent backwards on the cervix. Any combination of positions is possible. The retroverted, gravid (heavy or pregnant) uterus may possibly
impact in the bony pelvis at about the 12th week of pregnancy, and
happens if the fundus becomes wedged under the sacral promontory.

There is then no room in the pelvis for the bladder which becomes totally an abdominal organ, and the urethra is stretched considerably causing the patient to suffer from acute retention of urine. This impaction or incarceration of the uterus is not common and the patient is treated by slow decompression of the bladder by catheterization as she lies in a prone or semiprone position.

THE SUPPORTS OF THE UTERUS
The soft tissues that fill the outlet of the pelvis comprise the *pelvic floor*. In the erect attitude adopted by humans, the contents of the abdomen and pelvis rest upon the floor which thus of necessity needs to be strong. The floor is composed of skin, fat, muscle and connective tissue and contains apertures through which pass the rectum, vagina and urethra. The most important constituent is the musculature described below.

Study of Figures 10 and 11 show that in the female pelvis there is an area above the pelvic floor and below the reflection of the peritoneum. This area contains the pelvic fascia which invests the muscles and viscera and contains a loose connective tissue with fat which fills all the interstices in the pelvis. This zone of *pelvic cellular tissue* plays an important part in supporting the pelvic organs, acting in a manner that may be compared to the action of wood shavings used to protect glass or china when packed in a case. The tissue contains fibromuscular bands which help to support the uterus. These include the following three:

Transverse cervical ligaments
These pass from the side of the cervix to the side walls of the pelvis and are also known as Mackenrodt's ligaments.

Uterosacral ligaments
These pass backwards from the cervix on either side of the rectum and are attached to the front of the sacrum.

Round ligaments
These normally play little or no part in maintaining the position of the uterus but diverse surgical procedures have utilized them to antevert a uterus that is retrodisplaced (shortening the ligaments by plication, Gillam's operation, and the Baldy—Webster operation are but a few of the procedures described). However, these operations are performed much less frequently today than a generation ago. The round ligaments pass forwards and laterally from the body of the uterus just below and anterior to the insertion of the fallopian tubes. They pass through the inguinal canal via the deep inguinal ring and end by breaking up into strands which merge with the connective tissue in the labia majora.

Broad ligaments
Although these are mentioned here, they are not 'ligaments' but double folds of peritoneum draped over the tubes and passing from the margins of the uterus to the lateral walls of the pelvis.

The fascia and its areas of condensation or ligaments forms a continuous framework within the pelvis as stated earlier and one further condensation is to be noted. The *pubocervical* fascia extends from the transverse ligaments and passes anteriorly down the anterior vaginal wall beneath the base of the bladder to the body of the pubis. The integrity of this fascia is of some importance in supporting the bladder base and urethra.

The fallopian tubes
The fallopian tubes are two muscular ducts which transmit ova from the ovary to the uterine cavity. They extend laterally from the cornua of the corpus uteri towards the wall of the pelvis and are about 10 cm long. In the outer part of their course they curve backwards so that the extremity of each tube lies in the proximity of the ovary. The tubes are covered with the peritoneum of the broad ligaments except on the inferior aspects. The intermediate layer of involuntary muscle has external longitudinal and internal circular fibres and overlies a thin connective tissue submucous layer which contains the blood vessels and nerves supplying the mucous membrane. The latter inner layer con-

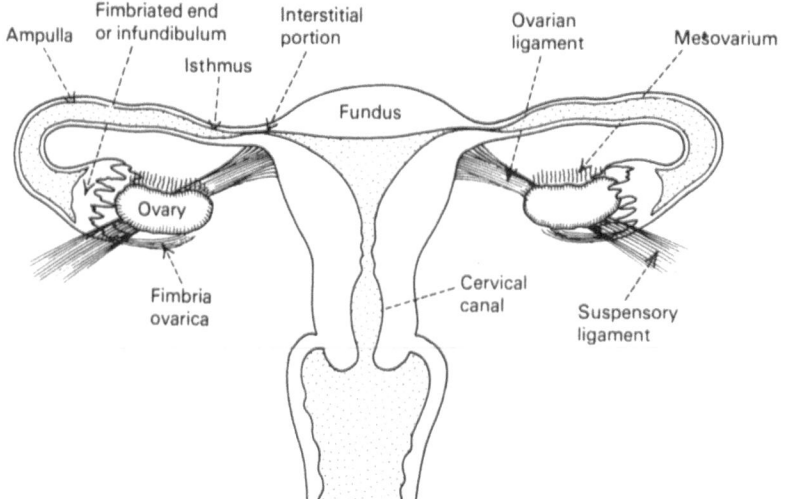

Figure 12 Posterial view of the uterus with fallopian tubes, ovaries and ligaments

sists of a columnar epithelium with many cells containing hair-like cilia that by their waving action set up a current, and this combined with tubal muscular peristaltic contractions may assist in propelling the ovum toward the uterine cavity. Cells with a secretive function are also present in the mucosa. The mucous membrane is thrown into a series of intricate longitudinal folds the pattern of which varies according to the location in the tube. Four areas of the tube are distinguished (Figure 12).

(1)   The *interstitial* portion. This is the part that passes through the wall of the uterus and is about 1 cm long.
(2)   The *isthmus* is the narrow third of the tube adjoining the uterus.
(3)   The *ampulla* is wider and comprises the majority of the tube.
(4)   The *fimbriated end* or infundibulum. The outer end of the tube is free of the enveloping broad ligament and has finger-like processes one of which is longer than the rest and extends to the ovary. The longer fimbria, the *fimbria ovarica*, is described as guiding the mature ovum into the tube at ovulation, and I have a mental picture of an elephant stuffing a bun into its mouth when describing this!

The ovaries
The ovaries are almond-shaped bodies approximately 3½ cm long, 2 cm wide and 1 cm thick. They normally lie high in the pouch of Douglas below the level of the fallopian tubes and are slung from the posterior layer of the broad ligament by a short peritoneal fold, the *mesovarium*. The blood vessels and nerves enter the anterior edge of the ovary at the *hilum*. The *ovarian ligament* attaches one end of the ovary to the uterus, while the other end is connected to the pelvic wall by a fold of peritoneum called the *suspensory* or *infundibulo-pelvic* ligament (Figure 12).

The ovary is covered by a membrane of low cuboidal cells, the *germinal epithelium*, so-called because it was considered that the oogonia or primordial ova originated from it. This is probably not so and their site of origin remains uncertain. The smooth glistening surface of the elongated ovary of the infant is not seen in the active gonad of the adult where the surface layer consists of an irregular pinkish-grey connective tissue sheet, the *tunica albuginea*.

The substance of the ovary may be divided into:

(1)   The outer *cortex* made up of the germinal epithelium and most of the many thousands of clusters of cells − the early or *primary*

follicles which are set in a dense framework of connective tissue, *the stroma.*
(2)   The inner *medulla,* which contains the supporting framework of connective tissue with most of the blood vessels and nerves of the ovary.

However, these two zones are not clearly defined. The development of the primary follicle is discussed in Chapter 2.

The musculature of the pelvic floor
The importance of the pelvic floor has already been mentioned when discussing the supports of the uterus (page 18). The muscles present are arranged in two layers:

(1)   An upper pair of strong muscles, the levatores ani, which are modified from those forming the tail muscles of animals.
(2)   A lower weaker system, which closes in the orifices of the pelvic outlet and forms an additional layer of muscle around the vagina.

THE LEVATORES ANI
These are two sheets of muscle which arise from the circumference of the true pelvis. Each muscle has a linear origin stretching from the back of the body of the pubis to the ischial spine. A study of a model

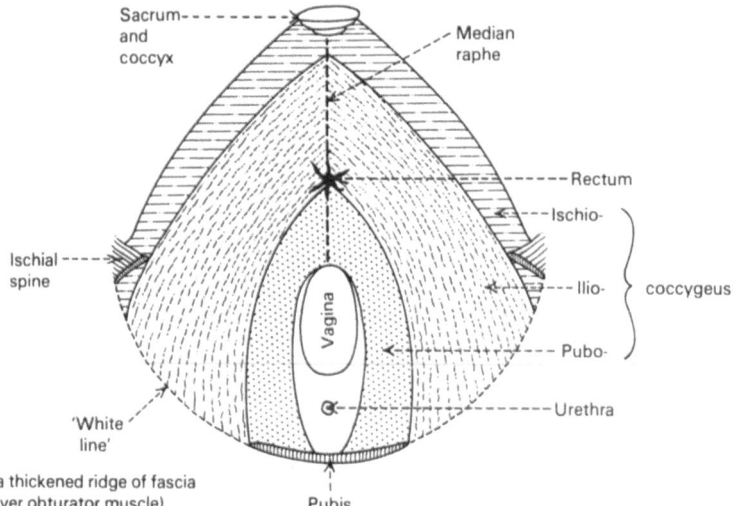

Figure 13   Schematic representation to show origin and insertion of levatores ani

pelvis will show that much of this zone is taken up by the aperture, the obturator foramen. This in life is covered by the thin obturator internus muscle which in turn is covered by fascia containing a thickened ridge called '*the white line*' from which the levatores ani arises. So the origin of each muscle is (a) from behind the pubis, (b) the 'white line', and (c) the ischial spine. The fibres then sweep downwards and medially across the pelvic outlet so that the upper surface of the muscle looks upwards, forwards and towards the midline. The posterior fibres (those arising from the ischial spine) come together on the sacrum and coccyx, while fibres from (b) and (c) meet in the midline or *median raphe* between coccyx and anus and perineum.

Because the muscles arise from areas of the pubis, ilium (white line) and ischium (the spine), the levatores ani are sometimes described as a muscular system consisting of pubo-, ilio- and ischio-coccygeus (Figure 13). I see no reason for this as the muscle acts as one entity and its contraction elevates both rectum and vagina. Furthermore, it acts as a sphincter constricting the lower ends of these passages.

THE SUPERFICIAL PERINEAL MUSCLES
These lie on the under-surface of the anterior part of the levatores ani in the pelvic outlet, surround the anal and vaginal orifices and form the superficial half of the muscles of the perineal body. The individual muscles that comprise this group are:

(1) The *transverse perinei* passing from perineum to ischial tuberosities.
(2) The *ischio-cavernosus* which extends from the ischial tuberosities to the clitoris.
(3) The *bulbo-cavernosus* which surrounds the vaginal orifice.
(4) The *external sphincter of the anus*.

The perineal body
This is a fibromuscular pyramid, the deeper part of which is formed by fibres of the levatores ani and the lower half by fibres of the superficial perineal muscles excluding the ischio-cavernosus. The relations of this structure are as shown in Figure 10.

The anatomy of labour
As the fetal head enters the pelvis, the bladder with its closely attached anterior vaginal wall is drawn upwards and forwards and the urethra is stretched almost to double its original length (from 4 cm to 8 cm). The posterior wall of the vagina and rectum and pelvic floor are pushed backwards and downwards and the pouch of Douglas is obliterated. As further descent of the fetus occurs the pelvic floor,

perineum and anus are stretched. The thick pyramidal perineal body becomes paper-thin.

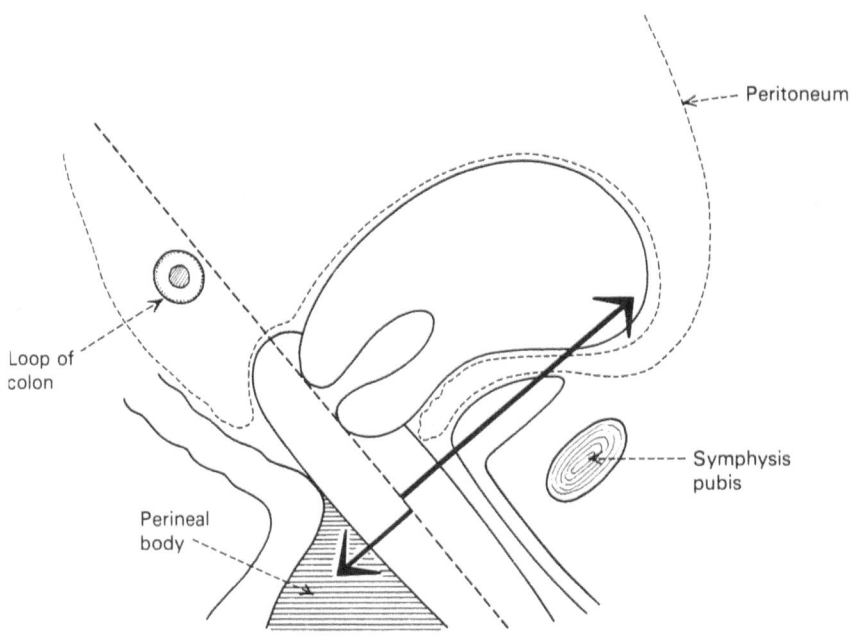

Figure 14 The anatomy of labour (see text)

The so-called anatomy of labour may be represented simply by referring to a lateral view diagram of the pelvis and drawing a line through the middle of the vagina parallel to its walls. As the fetus passes through the birth canal, the soft parts in front of the line are forced upwards and forwards, and those posterior to the line are pushed downwards and backwards (Figure 14).

2

Physiology

It was stated above that the sole function of the uterus is to receive, embed and nourish the fertilized ovum. To achieve these aims, every month during the child-bearing years the lining of the uterus, the endometrium, thickens and becomes filled with nourishing secretion. If pregnancy does not occur, menstruation follows in which the endometrium is shed. At the start of menstruation, the cycle and build-up of the endometrium recommences and preparations are again made to receive a possible pregnancy. How (and to a certain extent why) this occurs is discussed below under three separate headings:

(1) The cyclical changes that occur monthly in the ovary and the hormones involved.
(2) The effect that these hormones have upon the endometrium.
(3) The changes the ovum undergoes if fertilized, and how preparations are made for the fetus to embed and grow *in utero*.

It will thereafter be possible to correlate the various changes that take place.

Cyclical changes in the ovary
A summary of the cyclical changes in the ovary that normally occur in a fertile woman each month is

(1) The growth or maturation of the Graafian follicle.
(2) Ovulation.
(3) The formation of the corpus luteum.

THE MATURATION OF THE GRAAFIAN FOLLICLE
In the cortex of each ovary are found many thousands of clusters of cells, the early or primary follicles, containing the potential ova or oogonia in various stages of development. The derivation of the

24

various cells of the follicle may remain uncertain (see page 20) but the cyclical changes that occur in the follicle that will mature are best understood by visualizing the cellular cluster lying in and surrounded by the stroma. The cell earmarked to become the mature ovum of the month, grows much larger than the rest while some of the cytoplasm of the surrounding cells liquefies. This leaves a large cell (*the ovum*) amid a mass of others (the *discus proligerus* or *cumulus ovaricus*) at one end of the follicle, with a lining layer surrounding a drop of fluid – the *liquor folliculi*. The lining layer is but one or a few cells only in thickness, and as it has a granular appearance under the microscope is termed the *membrana granulosa*.

As the follicle matures, the stroma condenses around it to form an outer wall. The stroma adjacent to the membrana granulosa becomes vascular, while outside fibres increase in amount. Thus two covers encase the Graafian follicle, the *theca interna* (internal case) or *tunica vasculosa* (vascular coat) and the *theca externa* or *tunica fibrosa*.

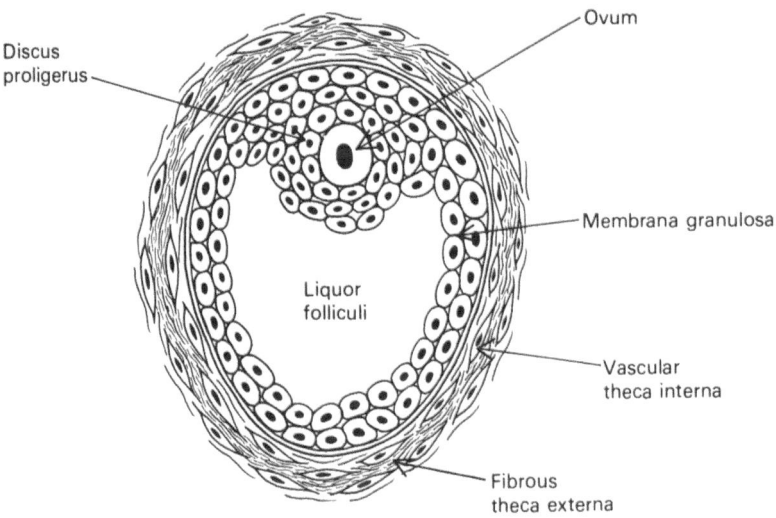

Figure 15   The mature Graafian follicle

OVULATION AND FORMATION OF THE CORPUS LUTEUM

The mature Graafian follicle is shown in Figure 15. The follicle increases in size and its walls thin as it reaches the surface of the ovary. Eventually the wall ruptures and the ovum surrounded by some cells of the discus is discharged into the peritoneum (ovulation) and taken into the fallopian tube. Rupture of the follicle is associated with bleeding into its cavity and the blood clot plugs the aperture. Immediately the cells of the membrana granulosa increase in size and number and a yellow material appears in the cytoplasm. Some cells from the theca interna similarly invade the clot. In this manner the yellow body or *corpus luteum* is formed.

If a pregnancy does not happen the corpus luteum begins to atrophy after about 10 days and is totally inactive just before the next menstruation. A microscopic white scar called the *corpus albicans* (white body) is left in the ovary. However, if the ovum is fertilized, the corpus luteum grows and remains active until the middle months of the pregnancy.

HORMONAL CONTROL

The cycle of events is controlled by hormones, and advances in the knowledge of this subject are made so rapidly today that most outside the specialized field of neuroendocrinology find difficulty in keeping up! A generation ago the anterior pituitary was considered to be the 'master gland', but for well over a decade it has been known that pituitary function is controlled by the hypothalamus. The latter secretes its own hormones and factors (which are agents known to be present but not yet fully identified or synthesized) and some of these stimulate the pituitary to increase its own hormone production in its turn. The interrelationship between the functions of the hypothalamus, pituitary and ovary is close, and mechanisms of control of menstruation are complex. Much is known about the pathways travelled by the various factors and also the so-called feedback mechanisms by which, for example, an increased production of oestrogens from the ovary effects the function of the hypothalamus and/or pituitary, but it is adequate in this study to note that the anterior pituitary hormone here concerned is called *gonadotrophin*, and its production is controlled by the *hypothalamic releasing hormone*. It has become fashionable to ease the complex matter by using the term *hypothalamic–pituitary axis* when discussing the control of the menstrual cycle! Indeed, suprathalamic factors including the cerebral cortex influence the axis, so that emotional upsets and drugs are among influences that may disturb the menstrual pattern.

Anterior pituitary gonadotrophin has two main constituents, *follicle-stimulating hormone* (FSH) and *luteinizing hormone* (LH). In the first half of the menstrual cycle FSH initiates and controls the maturation of the Graafian follicle which in its turn secretes *oestrogens*. In the middle of the menstrual month, ovulation occurs resulting in the formation of a corpus luteum. These latter changes are controlled by LH and the corpus luteum makes not only oestrogens but also *progesterone*. If pregnancy does not occur the corpus luteum dies, oestrogens and progesterone are withdrawn and menstruation follows. If, however, pregnancy takes place, the corpus luteum persists and increasing amounts of oestrogens and progesterone are liberated. The persistence of the corpus luteum in pregnancy may be due to a third constituent of the anterior pituitary gonadotrophin called luteotrophic hormone, but is more likely due to the hormones made by the trophoblast of the developing fetus. This hormone, called human chorionic gonadotrophin (HCG), is very similar to that made by the anterior pituitary gland and is discussed below (page 32).

Cyclical changes in the endometrium

When the Graafian follicle begins to ripen, the endometrium consists of a single layer of cubical epithelium with U-shaped dips passing through a connective tissue stroma to the muscle layer (myometrium). These straight narrow dips are termed *simple glands* even though no secretion is present. Between the glands lies the stroma containing spindle-shaped connective cells and some capillaries.

The maturing Graafian follicle manufacturing oestrogens causes the endometrium to thicken to a layer some 3 to 4 mm deep, as the glands elongate and become slightly tortuous, and the stroma cells and blood vessels multiply or proliferate. This is the *oestrogenic* or *proliferative phase*.

Then, after ovulation, the corpus luteum is formed and progesterone exerts its action on the endometrium already sensitized by oestrogens. The mucosa now thickens to a layer 6 to 7 mm in depth, the glands become extremely tortuous in their deeper parts and secretion appears in the cells and gland lumina. The stroma becomes oedematous as its cells multiply in size and number, and vascularity is markedly increased. These changes are more marked in the deeper layers of the endometrium which assumes a spongy appearance in this *progestational* or *secretory phase*.

If pregnancy does not occur the *menstrual phase* follows as a result of the withdrawal of oestrogens and progesterone associated with complete atrophy of the corpus luteum. In this phase most of the endometrium is shed, leaving behind the bases of the glands adjacent to the muscle layer. As menstruation continues, another follicle in the ovary begins to ripen, and from the cells left behind the endometrium regenerates and the cycle recommences (Figure 16).

DECIDUA FORMATION

If pregnancy occurs, secretory phase changes become more marked as glands become even more tortuous and vascularity increases. The stroma cells, now called *decidual cells*, become so numerous and large that they form almost a continuous sheet between the glands and

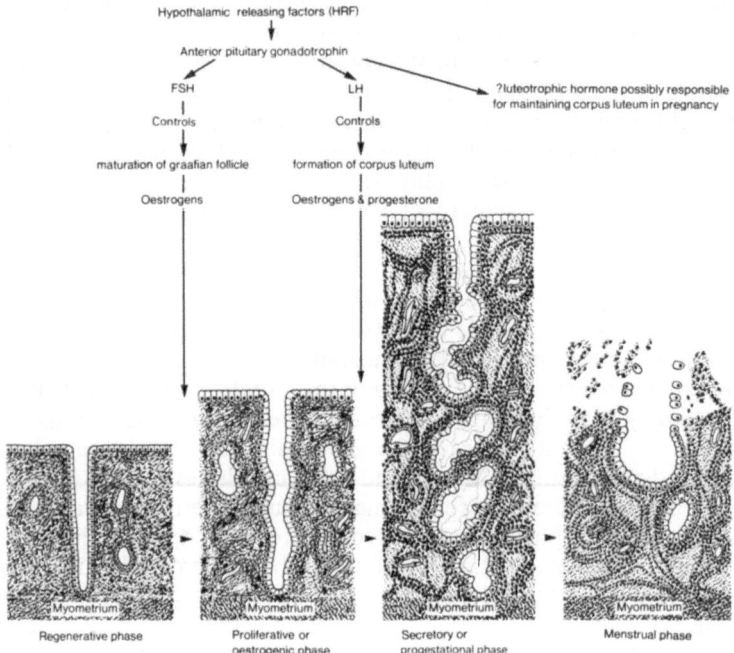

Figure 16 Control of menstrual cycle and cyclical changes in endometrium

blood spaces. The lining layer of the pregnant uterus is called the *decidua* although there is no marked difference between the decidua of early pregnancy and the endometrium of the non-pregnant uterus prior to menstruation – the difference is one of degree only. The exaggeration of the glandular and vascular spaces in the deeper layers of the decidua distinguishes:

(1) A superficial or compact layer.
(2) A deep spongy layer.
(3) A basal layer which is the base of the glands adjacent to the muscle layer or myometrium.

Fertilization and early development

Fertilization of the ovum occurs in the outer end of the ampulla of the fallopian tube. Pregnancy is initiated by the nucleus of a spermatozoon which has penetrated both cells of the discus and wall of the ovum, fusing with the nucleus of the latter to form the one-celled *zygote*, which commences mitotic division as it travels along the tube

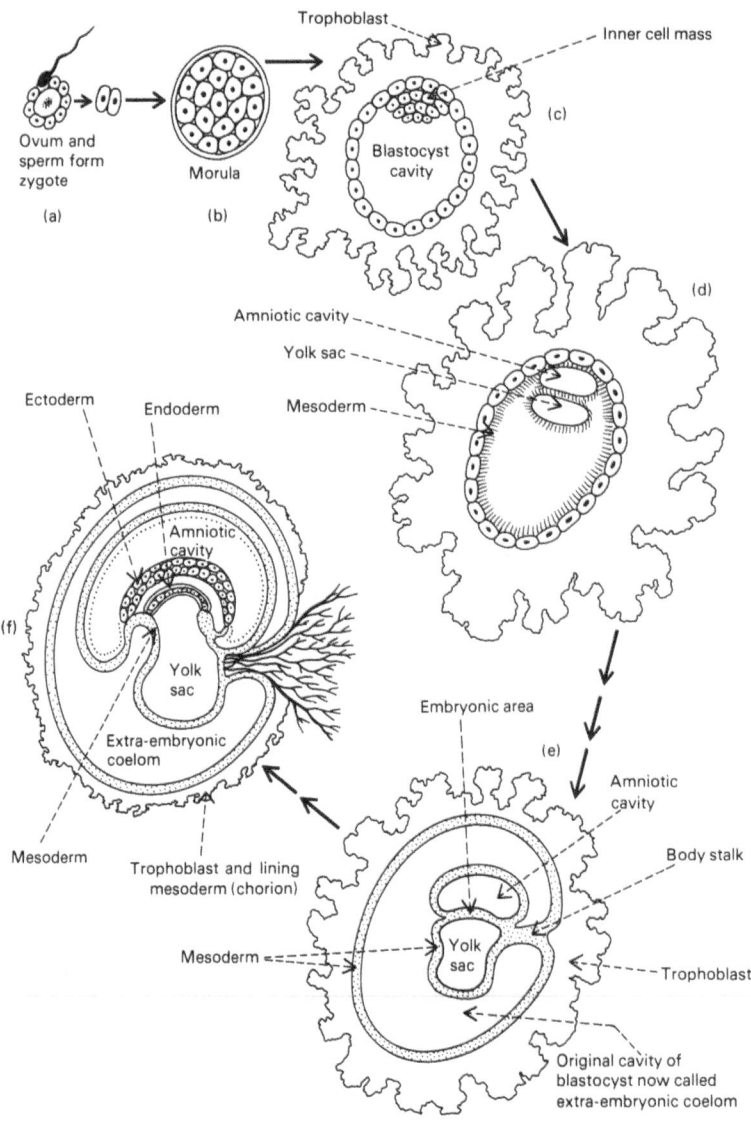

Figure 17   (a) to (f) early development of fetus

towards the uterine cavity. It divides into two *blastomeres*, then into four, eight and so on until a mulberry mass of cells called the *morula* is formed. The morula is not much bigger than the initial ovum as little nourishment is available from the endosalpinx. Indeed, if growth in size were excessive at this stage, the passage of the increasing cellular mass might become obstructed resulting in a tubal ectopic pregnancy.

When the morula enters the uterine cavity 5 or more days after ovulation, the surface cells differentiate from those in the centre to form the *trophoblast*, while within, a cavity, the *blastocoele*, appears leaving a cluster of cells at one pole. This cluster is the *inner cell mass*, and the whole structure is now the *blastocyst*. A few days later two cavities appear in the inner cell mass, the *amniotic cavity* and the *yolk sac*. The inner cell mass has become differentiated into two layers, the outer of *ectodermal cells* and the inner layer of smaller *endodermal cells* (Figure 17). During the next week the third primitive layer, the *mesoderm*, appears, as its cells fill the cavity of the blastocyst and condense to form a lining to the trophoblast and around the embryo and yolk sac. A band of mesodermal cells also insinuates itself between ectoderm and endoderm. It is from the small area where the three primitive layers meet, the *embryonic plate*, that the fetus is formed. The embryonic plate migrates towards the centre of the blastocyst and remains attached to the trophoblastic wall by the *body stalk* of mesoderm which later becomes the umbilical cord. As the amniotic cavity enlarges and fills with fluid, it surrounds the embryo.

A study of further development of the fetus requires textbooks devoted to the fascinating study of embryology. The ectoderm surrounds the other primitive layers and forms the skin and central nervous system. The endoderm forms the gut and the cells lining the glands that open into the alimentary canal (for example liver and pancreas) and most of the epithelium of the urinary bladder and urethra. From the mesoderm arise muscle, bone, blood and lymph vessels, connective tissue and most of the urogenital system. By the 8th week of pregnancy the embryo is recognizable as human. At 12 weeks, the fetus is 9 cm long with external ears, eyelids (fused until about the 6th month) and neck. Nails and external genitalia are beginning to appear. Sex may be determined from the latter during the following month.

THE TROPHOBLAST

It is now necessary to consider further the changes that are taking place in the outer layer of cells, the trophoblast. While the inner cell mass is forming, the trophoblast is pushing out processes which destroy the maternal endometrium and enable the growing mass to burrow into the decidua completely. (*Note*: The two terms 'endometrium' and 'decidua' have been used in one sentence especially to emphasize the fact that both terms indicate the lining mucosa of the uterus; endometrium is used in the non-pregnant state and decidua when pregnancy is present. As stated earlier, there is no qualitative difference between premenstrual endometrium and the decidua of early pregnancy.)

The outgrowths of trophoblast at an early stage of development divide into two layers (a) an inner cellular layer, the *cytotrophoblast* or *layer of Langhans*, and (b) an outer layer where the cell walls have disappeared to leave a multinucleated mass of cytoplasm called the *syncytiotrophoblast*. The syncytium elaborates enzymes which enable the outgrowths to burrow more and more deeply into the decidual glands and blood vessels. Although initially the trophoblastic outgrowths are solid structures they are soon penetrated by a core of mesoderm in which fetal blood vessels appear. In this way the *chorionic villi* are formed, and it should be noted that the blood systems of mother and fetus are always separated by the trophoblastic epithelium and mesoderm (Figure 18).

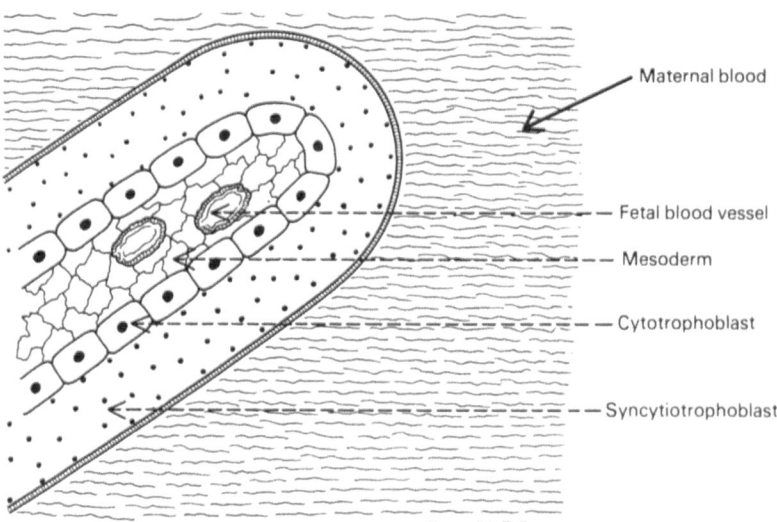

Figure 18   Schematic representation of a chorionic villus

FORMATION OF PLACENTA

Once the blastocyst has embedded completely into the decidua so rich in nutrients, it grows rapidly in size and as it extends into the uterine cavity three areas of the decidua become recognizable (Figure 19). The *decidua basalis* is the part that lies between the conceptus and the myometrium, while the *decidua capsularis* covers the area projec-

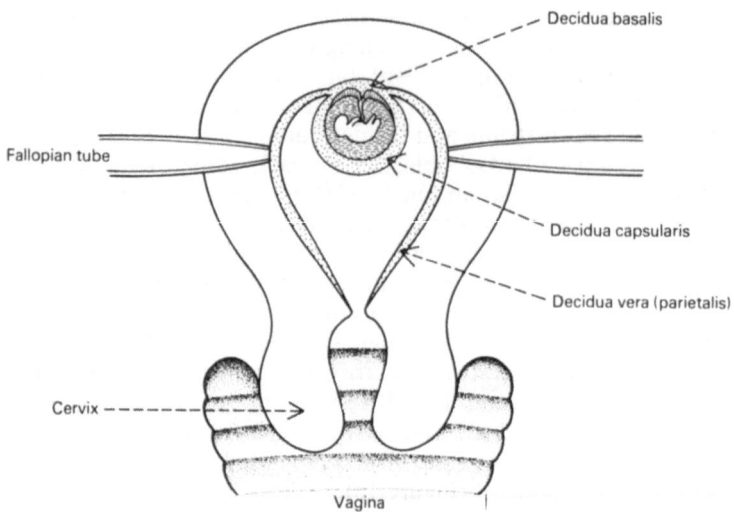

Figure 19   Decidual zones in early pregnancy

ting into the uterine cavity. The remainder is the *decidua vera* (decidua parietalis) the 'true' lining of the uterus. The growing fetal sac is at first surrounded by branching chorionic villi, but those in contact with the decidua capsularis begin to atrophy, and by the 12th week have formed the smooth *chorion laeve*. The villi in contact with the decidua basalis, however, continue to multiply and branch to form the very shaggy *chorion frondosum*. The placenta is formed from the latter and the decidua basalis, with maternal blood between the two. In the third stage of labour separation of the placenta takes place through the deep spongy layer of the decidua basalis, a zone which has been likened to the perforations separating stamps in a sheet.

At a very early stage in development the trophoblast elaborates a hormone similar to the anterior pituitary gonadotrophin. This is *human chorionic gonadotrophin* or HCG and, like that made by the anterior pituitary it contains both FSH and LH. HCG is probably responsible for the maintenance of the corpus luteum in pregnancy and may be found in both serum and urine. Its presence in the latter is utilized for pregnancy tests which are generally performed using immunological 'slide tests' some of which may give a reading within 2 minutes. The results are over 95 per cent accurate, and such tests in pregnancy should be positive 10 to 14 days after the first missed menstrual period.

Animals do not ovulate monthly but only at certain times (the period of oestrus or 'heat') and under the stimulus of copulation. This fact was utilized in earlier tests for pregnancy as ovulation would be stimulated if the animal were injected with urine containing HCG. Thus, virgin mice (Aschheim − Zondek) and rabbits (Friedman) were used and killed days after having received the injection. If the ovaries contained corpora lutea, the animal had ovulated and the test was positive. Later toads were utilized (Xenopus and Hogben tests). The female toad survived as she shed ova rather like frogspawn! Later it was found possible to utilize the male of the species in that sperms were shed and, indeed, the common or garden English frog was also of use (and much less expensive in the United Kingdom).

It should now be possible to correlate the various cyclical changes described. Each month a Graafian follicle matures, discharges an egg and the corpus luteum is formed. The hormones cause the endometrium to thicken and become secretory in readiness to receive the fertilized ovum. The latter, dividing in its journey along the fallopian tube, also elaborates enzymes to enable it to eat its way into the decidua. If pregnancy does not occur, the corpus luteum atrophies, oestrogens and progesterone are withdrawn, menstruation occurs and the cycle starts again.

MENSTRUATION

Menstruation itself is associated with changes in the hormone-sensitive blood vessels supplying the endometrium. The arterioles supplying the endometrium arise from a plexus of vessels in the muscular coat. Spiral arterioles grow from the basal to the superficial layer of the endometrium during the proliferative phase, and undergo spasmodic contractions, thereby cutting off the blood supply to the superficial parts of the endometrium. The mucosa blanches and degenerates and the glands empty as the endometrium shrinks.

When the vasoconstriction recedes, blood escapes through the walls of the blood vessels and haematomata form beneath the degenerating epithelium which is shed. Menstrual flow consists of blood and mucus, leukocytes and endometrial tissue and contains substances which can stimulate smooth muscle called *prostaglandins*. Menstrual blood does not normally clot in the vagina, probably because after clotting in the uterus it is liquefied by autolytic enzymes made by the degenerating endometrium.

It is of interest to note that the trophoblast, an actively growing structure, manufactures enzymes and erodes completely into the maternal tissues, very like the process of cancer. Yet in the vast majority of cases the placenta remains well localized and its formation causes no trouble. However, in the condition of proliferative hydatidiform mole (discussed in detail below, page 155), a complication of pregnancy, the fetus is blighted (does not develop) and the uterus becomes filled with actively growing chorionic villi which undergo cystic changes. The mole may eat its way completely through the wall of the uterus and secondary deposits appear in the lung. Yet the condition is innocent and there is some order to the pattern of growth. Indeed, in a normal pregnancy, trophoblastic cells enter the lungs and the appearance of secondary deposits is thus not necessarily evidence of malignancy. To take the process a stage further, however, when growth is completely without any order, the very malignant condition of chorioncarcinoma may occur. A generation ago this was invariably fatal, but now most cases are cured with cytotoxic drug therapy.

The exact nature of the mechanism which controls and localizes the placental development is unknown. Immunological and chemical factors are among those that remain subjects for research. A fibrinoid layer between trophoblast and decidua – the layer of Nitabuch – may be significant in this respect. In this era of advancement in techniques of organ transplants, the problems that arise because the recipient may reject foreign protein are not yet fully solved. Yet a mother does not usually reject the fetus *in utero* even though it may contain many substances foreign to her body. Although considerable research in autoimmunology has been done much remains to be done before the whole answer is obtained, and the placenta forms a fruitful ground for research.

Genetics

This is an appropriate time to consider some basic essentials of genetics. The living cell in its cytoplasm contains a membrane-bound nucleus within which may be found a nucleolus and various other intranuclear bodies. The important nucleic acid structure consists of *deoxyribonucleic acid* or *DNA*. This is associated with protein to form elongated threads – *the chromosomes*. The number of chromosomes in each cell is fixed for a given species and in the human being the number is 46; this number in each body or somatic cell is known as the *diploid number*. When a cell divides by *mitosis* (the usual division) the chromosomes split longitudinally so that each of the two cells formed retain 46. However, in the formation of the mature ovum or spermatozoon, *the gametes*, there is an atypical division – *meiosis* – in which the chromosomes instead of splitting form pairs, which then divide, half of each pair passing to one of the new cells formed and half to the other, so each cell has 23 chromosomes (*the haploid number*). When fertilization occurs and the zygote is formed by fusion of the two gametes, the diploid number 46 is restored.

The chromosomes in each gamete have their own shape and size, and like pairs with like in the formation of the zygote. The only pair that may not be identical are the sex chromosomes which are labelled X and Y. Thus, of the 46 chromosomes found in the normal somatic cell, 22 pairs consist of identical structures and the last pair may be XX (female) or XY (male). When meiosis occurs in the formation of the gamete, the mature ovum must contain the X chromosome, while the mature spermatozoon may contain either X or Y. When fertilization occurs, mathematically there is an equal chance that the zygote will thus contain XX or XY, a most convenient arrangement hopefully never to be disturbed by genetic engineers!

The carriers of genetic characteristics are *the genes* which are arranged in linear fashion, like beads on a string, each in a specified location or *locus*, on the chromosome. The locus is identical for corresponding genes in each of the pair of chromosomes (the pair consisting of one paternal and one maternal chromosome). Corresponding genes (called *alleles*) may be identical or not, and if different, may exhibit a dominant-recessive relationship. If the latter is the case, the specific characteristic carried by the dominant gene is shown and that of the recessive is not expressed.

In these days of advancing knowledge concerning the nature of the coded information carried by DNA, it is astonishing to think that over 115 years ago, a Moravian monk foretold the existence of genes which were either dominant or recessive, and propounded laws of heredity which are of import today. Gregor Johannes Mendel (1822–1884) experimented by cross-fertilizing peas, and the law of Mendelism was formulated in 1865. He crossed pure tall with pure dwarf peas, and the resultant generation appeared to be completely of tall peas. These, however, contained the recessive characteristic of dwarfness which was not expressed or which was masked, in other words, they were not pure but hybrid tall peas. When they were then crossed with each other, the resulting generation contained 1 in 4 dwarf peas (Figure 20).

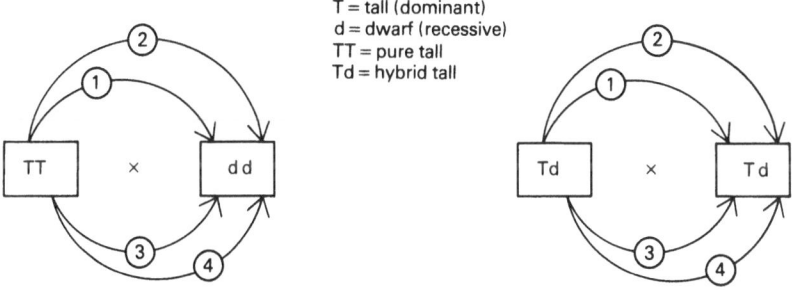

T = tall (dominant)
d = dwarf (recessive)
TT = pure tall
Td = hybrid tall

Figure 20   Mendelism, showing four possible results of cross-fertilization

If corresponding genes inherited from each parent are identical, the individual is pure for that characteristic and in humans the term used is *homozygous*. If, on the other hand, one gene is dominant and the other allele is recessive, the person is *heterozygous* for that factor.

3

Amenorrhoea: the diagnosis
and duration of pregnancy

In this chapter the features that lead to the diagnosis of pregnancy and help to determine the estimated date of delivery (EDD) are discussed. As many of the signs and symptoms are only presumptive evidence of pregnancy while others are positive indicators of the condition, it is a worthwhile exercise here to consider which is which. The words 'signs' and 'symptoms' incidentally should not be confused – signs are elicited on examination by a trained person, but the patient experiences symptoms.

Amenorrhoea
Cessation of menstruation is usually the first symptom that alerts a woman to the fact that she may be pregnant, but there are numerous other causes of amenorrhoea, which may be primary or secondary, and physiological or pathological.

PHYSIOLOGICAL AMENORRHOEA
This is present during the following three stages of life.

(1) Before the menarche (the onset of menses).
(2) During pregnancy and the puerperium and, to a variable degree, during lactation.
(3) After the menopause, a condition associated with diminished ovarian hormone production.

PATHOLOGICAL AMENORRHOEA
This may be due to

(1) *Hormonal disturbances* which originate anywhere in the hypothalamic–pituitary–ovarian axis. Organs such as the thyroid and the cortex of the adrenal gland may also affect the function of the axis and lead to amenorrhoea. The ovaries possess a very high

reserve capability and a woman can function quite normally if left with even less than a half of one ovary. However, ovarian causes of secondary amenorrhoea include the polycystic ovarian syndrome (*Stein—Leventhal syndrome*), virilizing tumours and malignancies. Ovarian failure at an early age is occasionally associated with sex chromosome anomalies, and sometimes there is no apparent reason for a very early menopause.

(2)   *Unreactive endometrium.* Amenorrhoea may be associated with a normal hormone status and the fault may lie in the 'target' at which the hormones are aimed, that is the endometrium which fails to react. Examples of this are seen in tuberculous endometritis and in a condition of endometrial sclerosis which may follow excessively vigorous curettage (*Asherman's syndrome*).

(3)   *General diseases* which include uncontrolled diabetes mellitus, pulmonary tuberculosis and any pyrexial condition.

Suprathalamic causes of amenorrhoea

A group of causes of amenorrhoea which has not been included under the heading of hormonal disturbances (see (1) above) are now listed individually. They are important and not uncommon. They may act by depressing the hypothalamus or inhibiting the production of its releasing factor (page 26) and are thus sometimes referred to as being suprathalamic in origin.

(1)   Emotional strain such as domestic crisis or tragedy, moving house, changing occupation or taking an important examination.

(2)   *Pseudocyesis* (the 'phantom' pregnancy) which in my experience is more often associated with the desire for, rather than the fear of, a pregnancy. Other features of pregnancy also show in this condition including breast changes and increasing abdominal girth, and patients may state with conviction that they feel fetal movements. Doctors and nurses may be unaware of the 'pseudo' nature of the pregnancy for months.

(3)   *Malnutrition*, possibly self-imposed because of over-enthusiastic dieting, or associated with psychiatric disturbance as in the syndrome of *anorexia nervosa*. Insufficient calorie intake can cause amenorrhoea before any other effect on bodily health is shown.

(4)   *Drugs* such as chlorpromazine (Largactil) and certain hypotensive reagents may depress the hypothalamus.

Oral contraceptives may be included under the heading *iatrogenic* (produced by the physician) causes. I have examined scores of women who fail to menstruate normally for many months when they stop taking the Pill and found the uterus to be smaller than usual. If a year after ceasing hormonal contraceptive therapy normal menstruation has not recommenced the patient needs gynaecological investigation.

Diagnosis of pregnancy
UTERINE GROWTH

After the sixth week of pregnancy the uterus begins to enlarge, soften and becomes globular. Many textbooks describe *Hegar's sign* which is stated to be positive between the 8th and 12th week of pregnancy. Hegar's sign is elicited on bimanual examination at which the doctor should appreciate a globular fundus and, because the uterus is softened and not yet filled with the developing pregnancy, the internal and external fingers may meet in the region of the isthmus (Figure 21). I do not think that this sign should be looked for to diagnose early pregnancy, and attempts to elicit it by other than the most gentle of examiners might well be classified with abortifacients!

After the 12th week of pregnancy the uterus rises out of the pelvis, becomes an abdominal organ and may be palpated suprapubically. At about 20 weeks the organ is at the level of the umbilicus, and at 36 weeks the xiphisternum is reached. Thereafter the level may drop slightly (the patient experiences 'lightening') as the fetal head enters the pelvis. The times given are only approximate but are initially useful guides to practitioners. Estimates of the duration of pregnancy by abdominal palpation become more accurate with experience.

In the last trimester (3 months) of pregnancy, the uterus may be felt to be contracting rhythmically. These are the so-called *Braxton–Hicks* painless contractions and the patient should be unaware of their existence. This is not invariably so, but if the contractions are associated with marked discomfort, one should consider that the onset of labour is imminent.

EVIDENCE OF THE FETUS

The earliest evidence of the presence of a fetus in utero is obtained by ultrasonic echogram and specialists in the technique are able to detect this at about 6 weeks. Clinically, and without these more sophisticated aids, the presence of a fetus cannot be determined before 16 weeks.

Ballottement
The fetus lies in its bag of amniotic fluid, and pressure applied evenly, sharply but gently with the fingertips may cause it to move away and then float back to impinge on the finger-tips. If pressure is applied internally, usually through the anterior fornix, this *internal ballottement* is positive after the 16th week of pregnancy. *External ballottement* by

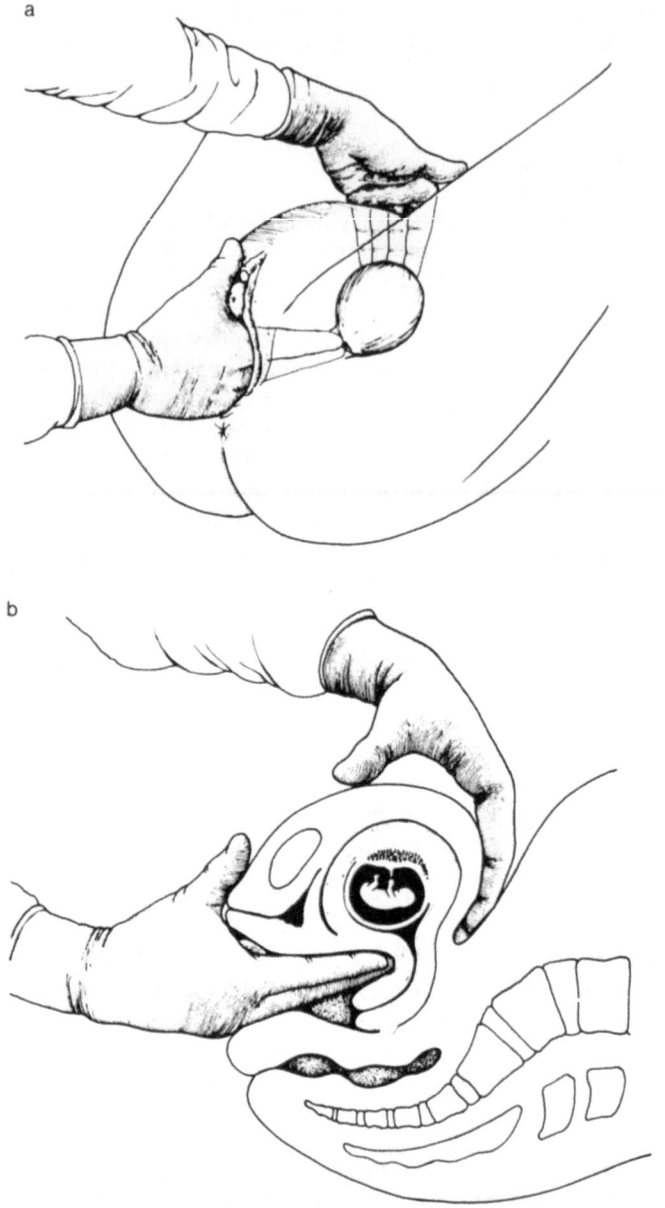

Figure 21   Hegar's sign (a) Palpating the globular uterus; (b) Examining hands
may almost meet at level of isthmus. See text

which pressure is applied via the abdominal wall is not positive until after the 18th week.

Fetal heart sounds

These are detectable at or shortly after the 12th week of pregnancy with relatively simple and portable ultrasonic machines. For this investigation the patient should have a full bladder (this is almost unique for all other examinations in obstetrics and gynaecology). With ordinary stethoscopes or with the naked ear the fetal heart cannot usually be heard until after 20 weeks. In the last trimester of pregnancy the fetal heart, best heard generally over the back of the fetus, beats at a rate varying between 120 and 160 per minute.

Sometimes during auscultation a blowing sound is detected and this is called a *souffle*. The *funic souffle* is due to the blood rushing through the umbilical arteries and thus its rate is that of the fetal heart. A loud *uterine souffle* may also be heard as the blood flows through the hypertrophied tortuous uterine blood vessels, and the rate of this corresponds with the maternal heart or pulse.

The time at which the mother first feels *fetal movements* is very variable indeed. For purposes of calculating the EDD, I consider the primigravida feels movements ('quickening') at 19 weeks and the multigravida at 18 weeks. However, many women who have had children have convinced me that they have felt fetal movements as early as 15 weeks.

Although X-rays can provide evidence of fetal bones at 15 weeks such investigation is contraindicated in a normal continuing pregnancy. In fact, X-ray investigation should always be kept to a minimum and performed only in the last weeks of pregnancy.

Breast changes

A patient may complain of heaviness and a tingling sensation in the breasts even before missing her first menstrual period, but premenstrual tension is no rarity and many women have these symptoms even when not pregnant. The areola around the nipple enlarges and darkens, and sebaceous areolar glands become more prominent (*Montgomery's tubercles*), signs which are more significant in blonde primigravidae. The vascularity of the breasts increases and veins become more prominent (infrared photography shows this and a few decades ago this was suggested as a possible diagnostic aid in pregnancy!) A colourless fluid may be expressed from the nipples at 12 weeks, and a turbid *colostrum*, the precursor of milk, at 16 weeks. True milk secretion does not start until a few days after the birth of the baby.

'Morning sickness'

Nausea, with or without vomiting, is fairly common in early pregnancy and may affect nearly 50 per cent of all women from about the 6th to the 16th week of pregnancy. The disturbance does not necessarily occur in the morning and all grades of severity are met, from mild transient nausea to a serious condition that can jeopardize the patient's life. The subjects of nausea and hyperemesis gravidarum (excessive vomiting in pregnancy) are dealt with in Chapter 16.

Pressure symptoms

Day frequency of micturition is very common, occurs from the 6th to the 12th week of pregnancy, and often indicates that the uterus is in the normal position of anteversion and anteflexion. At 6 weeks the uterus is becoming globular and enlarging so that it presses on the bladder when the patient is in the erect posture. At night and in bed this pressure is removed. At 12 weeks when the uterus rises out of the pelvis into the abdomen, the pressure is relieved and the symptom disappears.

Some patients, however, have frequency of micturition throughout the pregnancy. This may be a physiological phenomenon associated with increased fluid intake, the latter presumably caused by pregnancy stimulating the hypothalamus which possesses a 'thirst or drinking' centre!

Other pressure symptoms that occur later in pregnancy (by which time one hopes the condition has been diagnosed) include varicose veins and haemorrhoids, constipation and heartburn. The latter occurs in the last weeks of pregnancy when the uterus has extended into the upper abdomen, presses on the stomach and causes its acid contents to be regurgitated into the oesophagus. Considerable relief may be obtained by advising the patient not to lie too flat (use an extra pillow or two) and take a simple antacid.

Progesterone, essential for the maintenance of pregnancy in animals, relaxes smooth muscle and by exerting this action upon gut, blood vessels, cardiac sphincter of the stomach and ureters has been blamed for constipation, varicosities, heartburn and hydro-ureter respectively. The fact that non-pregnant women on progesterone therapy do not develop these symptoms has led many to question this villainous role of progesterone!

Increased vascularity of the vagina and cervix in pregnancy is associated with increasing amounts of circulating oestrogens. These areas soften and develop a violet tinge in the first trimester.

The fact that progesterone raises the basic body temperature is utilized in subfertility investigations and family planning to establish whether there is ovulation. A woman who records her temperature – 3 minutes by the clock is the *minimum* time required for recording basic temperature orally – usually finds that there is a rise of 0.2 °C or more following ovulation and that the temperature falls as menstruation commences. If she becomes pregnant, the elevated temperature will persist. However excessive use of temperature recording in subfertility investigations is undesirable as it often has adverse psychological effects.

Pregnancy tests
These have been discussed (page 32). They depend upon the presence of human chorionic gonadotrophin (HCG) in the urine and should give positive results within 2 weeks of the first missed period. The immunological slide tests are the most widely used and results are obtained within a few minutes. Manufacturers supply simple instructions with kits sold in the United Kingdom but tests are better performed by trained technicians. The administration of any form of hormone as a test for pregnancy is contraindicated as the fetus may be adversely affected.

Estimated date of delivery (EDD)
For about 300 years, or a century before Franz Carl Naegele was born in Düsseldorf, Germany, the 'rule' that bears his name has been used for calculating the EDD. By this rule, 7 days are added and 3 months deducted from the first day of the last menstrual period (LMP) to obtain the date when the fetus may be considered fully mature. It is a very simple procedure and one I have always used. If, for example, the LMP commenced for instance on 14 June, the 6th month, the EDD is then the 21st day of the 3rd month, or March. I find sometimes that there is a little hesitancy when the LMP was towards the end of January, February or March, but there is no need for confusion if one counts these as the 13th, 14th and 15th months; so, if the LMP started on 26 February (26.14), by adding 7 days and deducting 3 months the EDD is 33 November, in other words 3 December.

If one makes small allowances for the variation in the number of days in each month, the total time from LMP to EDD is 280 days. The period of *gestation* (or 'carrying') commences from the time of fertilization of the ovum and this will be approximately 14 days less. Ovulation, however, varies quite considerably (even in a woman with a most regular cycle) so at best the date recorded for delivery is only an estimate.

There are many causes for error in arriving at the EDD.

(1)   Patient error or ignorance of dates.
(2)   An error in calculation by doctor or midwife.
(3)   An irregular menstrual cycle in which the day of ovulation may be grossly miscalculated.
(4)   Pregnancy occurring after the use of oral contraceptives; ovulation in the initial months after stopping these hormones may be delayed and this is now a common cause for recording an incorrect EDD.
(5)   During lactation, when ovulation is very variable, menstruation may be suppressed for a time; prolactin production is high and gonadotrophin levels low. It is not uncommon for pregnancy to occur before menstruation recommences after parturition.
(6)   A threatened abortion, or decidual bleeding which may cause blood loss at the time of the missed periods up to the 12th week of pregnancy, may be mistaken for normal menstruation (see page 149).
(7)   Other causes of amenorrhoea, such as emotional upsets, and those discussed above.

Intrauterine fetal death
If the fetus dies in utero in the second half of pregnancy, signs and symptoms of pregnancy that have been present will retrogress. The uterus ceases to grow and may become smaller, fetal movements cease and heart sounds are absent. These features may be demonstrated by ultrasonic echogram, and X-ray evidence of intrauterine death is present 10 or more days after its occurrence. *Spalding's sign* is positive when considerable overlapping of the fetal skull bones is shown, associated often with acute flexion of the spine.

In earlier pregnancy a dead fetus is sometimes retained in utero when the diagnosis is one of *missed abortion*. This may be preceded by a threatened abortion with associated vaginal bleeding or brown discharge, but sometimes there are no vaginal losses. Pregnancy tests become negative within a week of intrauterine death and oestriols disappear from the urine (see page 190). A *carneous mole*, so-called because of its fleshy appearance, is a missed abortion in which the fetus has been killed by repeated haemorrhages into the chorionic—decidual space. The wall of the mole consists of layers of blood clot which surround a collapsed amniotic sac containing the blighted fetus. The latter may present as a small white speck only. The treatment of missed abortion is to evacuate the uterus either surgically or by oxytocic drugs. These subjects are discussed below (Chapter 17).

Finally it is worthwhile noting that all the following conditions have been mistaken for pregnancy.

    (1)   Fat
    (2)   Flatus
    (3)   Fluid, that is ascites
    (4)   Full bladder
    (5)   Fibroids
    (6)   False pregnancy − pseudocyesis
    (7)   Ovarian cysts.

4

Prenatal care

The aims of prenatal care

The purpose of prenatal care is to ensure that a woman remains as fit, healthy and content as possible and has a healthy baby in the easiest and happiest manner. To achieve this, other factors are essential in addition to regular prenatal checks.

Confidence is of prime importance – confidence in herself and in the midwife. *Knowledge* helps to build confidence, and while it is unnecessary for the patient to study textbooks concerning childbirth and baby care, which could in fact be unsettling, some selected literature may be of value. Thus each expectant mother at my units is presented with a booklet giving information about the hospital, the facilities and staff, and the various classes held. It also contains brief advice on many topics including diet (see below page 47). However, the most important method of obtaining knowledge and building confidence is the direct contact between patient and practitioner. After each and every prenatal consultation I invariably tell the patient all is well (if it is) and invite questions.

Preparation for childbirth takes the form of supervised exercises including breathing. 'Relaxation exercises' are aimed primarily at giving the patient confidence in herself during the first stage of labour when she may not always have trained staff with her. Authorities differ in the methods used. The popular term 'psychoprophylaxis' is used for a method in which a pattern of breathing exercises is followed. This, accompanied by light stroking massage applied to back or abdomen (effleurage) may help condition a woman psychologically for labour. In the past various devices such as negative pressure bags and chairs have been recommended, and doubtless are still being used in some centres though many may question their value. Any method or exercise which helps the patient to gain confidence, provided it is in no way harmful, must be considered of value.

Diet
The booklet issued to women at their first prenatal visit (mentioned above) states:

'As a general rule you may have all the things you are accustomed to eating. In pregnancy, however, because of the extra needs of your body and of the baby, the following guiding principles should be observed.

(1) Starchy foods such as bread, potatoes and sugar should be taken only in moderation. Avoid also an excessive amount of salt.
(2) The body-building proteins such as meat, fish, eggs and cheese are good for you, as are also fresh fruit and green vegetables.
(3) At least one pint, and preferably two pints of milk should be taken daily. Drink as much as you feel like drinking, but it is unnecessary to drink large quantities of fluid. Alcohol, certainly in large quantities, should be avoided.
(4) You will be given iron tablets to take during the pregnancy.'

Nutrition in pregnancy is of great importance, as it supplies energy and maintains body tissues. The fetus, of course makes nutritional demands on the mother, but she does not need to 'eat for two' as there is only a slight rise in the daily calorie requirement. In the United Kingdom malnutrition is rare, but in many areas of the world this is not so. Maternal malnutrition is associated with a markedly increased maternal and perinatal mortality (stillbirths and deaths in the first week of life).

BODY REQUIREMENTS
In addition to the three main classes of food, carbohydrates, proteins and fats, the body requires minerals such as calcium (Ca), potassium (K), sodium (Na), magnesium (Mg), phosphorus (P) and iron (Fe) and vitamins.
  Carbohydrates are the main source of supply for energy used in physical activity including that of labour. *Proteins*, which are composed of numerous amino-acids, are necessary for 'body-building' not only because the fetus and placenta are growing but also because tissue breakdown and formation is a continuous process in the human body. First-class proteins such as meat, fish, eggs and milk contain all the essential amino-acids, some of which may be lacking in the important *nutritive* group of second-class proteins (vegetable proteins in cereals and pulses). *Fats* or lipids provide the main source for storing energy. If carbohydrate supplies are inadequate, fats may be utilized but they

cannot be completely oxidized into fatty acids. The process stops short at the stage in which acetone and acetoacetic acids are produced and these substances are found in the urine when the patient is in a state of ketoacidosis (acetoketosis).

Mineral deficiency, apart from that of iron, is rare in the United Kingdom. Calcium requires sufficient vitamin D to be absorbed adequately and lack of these substances may be associated with osteomalacia and rickets – diseases rarely encountered in the United Kingdom, but still found in parts of India and Pakistan, especially in multipara whose calcium intake is inadequate. A minimum of one pint of milk daily as recommended in (3) above provides the calcium required in pregnancy. Maternal iodine deficiency causing fetal goitre and cretinism is still endemic in parts of the Third World.

Vitamins, substances essential for life (although not all are amines as originally thought), are divided into those that are (a) *fat soluble* – A, D, E, and K (lack of vitamin K in the newborn may be associated with haemorrhage), and (b) *water soluble* – the B complex group and vitamin C. Vitamin B_1 or thiamine was thought to be a factor in causing pre-eclampsia. Vitamin C is found in citrus fruits and green vegetables, and even though boiling greens effectively destroys all the vitamin C content, diseases like scurvy are almost unknown in the West.

Halibut (or cod) liver oil, a popular method of giving additional fat-soluble vitamins is nowadays rarely necessary in the United Kingdom.

Frequency of prenatal consultations
A woman should be seen by her doctor in the first 12 weeks of her pregnancy. Thereafter examination is performed every 4 weeks until the 28th week, then fortnightly to 36 weeks and weekly in the last month. This assumes that pregnancy lasts 40 weeks (an estimation only, see page 43) and constitutes the minimal safe care. More frequent checks are often necessary and it is of vital (in its literal sense) importance to ensure that there is the closest cooperation between hospital specialists, general practitioners and nurses, all of whom may be involved in looking after the expectant mother. Unhappily it may be lack of cooperation from the mother herself which can lead to tragedy.

The first examination
It is essential to record accurately the woman's history, the findings at each examination and her complaints (if any) with advice given and treatment prescribed. The following are of importance.

(1) Personal data.
(2) Menstrual history. Are menstrual periods regular? Was the last menstrual period (LMP) normal in time, behaviour and duration? Are there any other possible causes for amenorrhoea? (page 37).
Has there been any vaginal bleeding or discharge since the LMP?
(3) The estimated date of delivery (EDD) as calculated from the first day of the LMP.
(4) Previous obstetric history. All previous pregnancies should be noted in chronological order with particular attention being given to:

(a) The duration of the pregnancy.
(b) The occurrence of any complications during the prenatal period.
(c) The duration of labour and the mode of delivery − whether labour was induced or delivery assisted.
(d) Was there any postpartum haemorrhage, or infection?
(e) The sex and weight of the baby and its condition at birth.
(f) Were sutures necessary?
(g) Was the baby breast fed, and if so, for how long, and is the baby well now?

(5) Previous medical history and family history. Special attention is paid to any condition that may be associated with cardiac complications, although the incidence of rheumatic heart disease in pregnancy has diminished considerably due largely to the effective treatment of streptococcal infections and rheumatic fever in childhood. Previous virus infections (including rubella), episodes of venous thrombosis, upper respiratory and urinary tract infections and kidney disease are noted, as well as surgical operations and whether or not the patient has had a blood transfusion. A personal or family history of diabetes, tuberculosis, hypertension, multiple pregnancy or congenital abnormality may be significant. A record is made of any known allergies, and of any drugs the patient may be taking.

The first physical examination by the doctor includes at least that of heart, lungs, breasts, abdomen and pelvis. In addition to blood pressure and urine analysis, a record is made of height, weight, presence or absence of varicosities and of any deformity or abnormality in general configuration. Vaginal examination and pelvic assessment (page 5) should usually be performed at the initial examination. It is sometimes stated that internal examination is better deferred until the last trimester of pregnancy because the patient knows her doctor better and has more confidence, and as the pelvic floor is softer deeper palpation is possible which enables a better clinical estimation of the true pelvis. This is certainly correct, but I think that the experienced practitioner should be able to instil confidence in most patients at the first meeting. If, however, a miscarriage occurs within a few weeks of a pelvic examination being carried out the doctor may be blamed for this. Certainly in a patient with a history of previous abortion or recent blood loss, the examination may be deferred.

I consider early vaginal examination preferable because:

(1)   Estimation of uterine size and duration of pregnancy is more accurate in the first 3 to 4 months.
(2)   The position of the uterus is ascertained.
(3)   Uterine and ovarian pathology may be excluded.

If the uterus is retrodisplaced it is possible that there is a minimal increase in the risk of miscarriage, but attempts to correct the position are more likely to cause trouble: I reassure the patient that all is well but tell her that her uterus is 'tilted backwards', a common finding, and advise her to:

(1)   Not indulge in strenuous exercise.
(2)   Abstain from coitus especially when her periods would have been due.
(3)   Occasionally adopt the prone attitude in bed, which will help the uterus come forward but need be adopted only when the patient wishes and as long as no discomfort occurs.

These minor precautions should be taken until the 14th week of pregnancy by which time the uterus should have risen well into the abdomen and thus cannot retrovert again; also the placenta will be well formed diminishing the danger of miscarriage. Acute retention of urine resulting from impaction of the markedly retroverted and retroflexed uterus at about the 12th week of pregnancy is rare, so it is only seldom necessary for the patient to seek medical advice if there are difficulties in micturition.

Blood tests and screening techniques
Tests on blood obtained by venepuncture are performed at the first visit and include:

(1) Haemoglobin level and packed cell volume (pcv), and where possible a full blood picture.
(2) ABO group and rhesus factor; Rh antibody screening tests.
(3) Haemoglobin electrophoresis for abnormal haemoglobins where applicable.
(4) Serology to exclude syphilis by VDRL slide test and TPHA. The Wassermann and Kahn tests are now considered obsolete in the United Kingdom but may still be applicable in some areas.
(5) Rubella antibody tests. This screening test is performed on all patients in my units. If the titre is 1 in 16 or less the patient is considered 'at risk' and this fact is recorded. She is offered active immunization which will be given to her if she so desires on the first day after delivery. Rubella vaccine (Almevax 0.5 ml) is given subcutaneously and the patient is warned to avoid pregnancy for the next 3 months. She is also offered an intramuscular injection of medroxyprogesterone-acetate (Depoprovera 150 mg) as a short-term contraceptive measure, but I am not a keen advocate of this as several patients have complained of slight but prolonged vaginal bleeding which may be associated with the hormone.
(6) Screening for anencephaly and spina bifida by measuring the concentration of alphafetoprotein in maternal serum is of some value. If the serum levels are raised, ultrasonography and amniocentesis are undertaken.

(1) and (2) above are discussed further in Chapter 5 on anaemias.

Where there are facilities for *ultrasonography*, some experts in this field consider it desirable for all expectant mothers to undergo screening. The echogram is of special value in detecting:

(1) Early pregnancy (both intrauterine and extrauterine)
(2) Certain fetal abnormalities at an early stage, such as spina bifida
(3) Multiple pregnancy
(4) Molar pregnancy
(5) The placental site
(6) Fetal maturity, which may be estimated especially in mid-pregnancy
(7) Intrauterine growth which may be monitored by serial scanning.

Furthermore, the boost given to the mother's morale in seeing her baby move is often considerable. As yet no harmful effects to the fetus have been demonstrated, but personal preference is for selective use of ultrasonography.

Amniocentesis
This procedure is one in which a sample of amniotic fluid is removed by passing a needle into the uterus usually via the abdominal wall, and is a useful screening for detecting:

(1)   Certain neural tube defects (by estimating alphafetoprotein levels).
(2)   Certain chromosomal abnormalities such as Down's syndrome (mongolism).
(3)   The degree of Rh isoimmunization by spectrophotometric estimation of bilirubin levels.
(4)   Fetal maturity.
(5)   The sex of the fetus (structures called Barr bodies are looked for in the nuclei of cultured cells from the amniotic fluid; this may be important when certain inherited sex-linked conditions are under consideration).

Amniocentesis, however, is not without risk, such as inducing labour prematurely, haemorrhage, or introducing infection, so it is not undertaken without good cause. The overall risk of the procedure is in the region of 1%.

SUBSEQUENT EXAMINATIONS
At each subsequent prenatal examination the patient is weighed, blood pressure checked and a clean specimen of urine is tested for protein, sugar and acetone. The abdomen is palpated to ascertain whether the uterus and fetus are growing as anticipated and legs and hands are examined for oedema. The date on which fetal movements were first felt by the expectant mother is recorded, and in the second half of the pregnancy the fetal heart is checked at every examination. Any complaints are discussed and recorded. The significance of all these features is considered in the relevant chapters below, but accurate records are particularly essential when prenatal examinations may not always be performed by the same practitioner.

Abdominal palpation
This is helped if the patient is relaxed and the examiner has warm hands and short rounded fingernails. The importance of confidence has been stressed, and if the woman is lying on a firm couch (which is to be preferred) the abdominal muscles are more relaxed when she bends her knees fractionally and breathes quietly through the mouth with the head to one side.
The examiner (certainly if right-handed) stands to the patient's right

and first feels the fundus to estimate the size of the uterus. In the last 2 months of pregnancy the fetal position should be determined, noting in order:

(1) The fetal *lie* − which expresses the relationship between the longitudinal axis of the fetus and that of the uterus; the lie is longitudinal, oblique or transverse.

(2) The *presentation* − which nominates the part of the fetus lying over the internal os. If the fetal head presents (cephalic presentation) its *attitude* is determined. This is normally one of flexion in which case the vertex is the presenting part. If the head is extended, the presentation may be either a face (full extension) or brow (partial extension).

(3) The *position* indicates more precisely the relationship between the presenting part and the maternal pelvis. To ascertain the position an arbitrary bony point of the fetus called the *denominator* is related to the nearest one of six points on the maternal pelvic inlet (Figure 22).

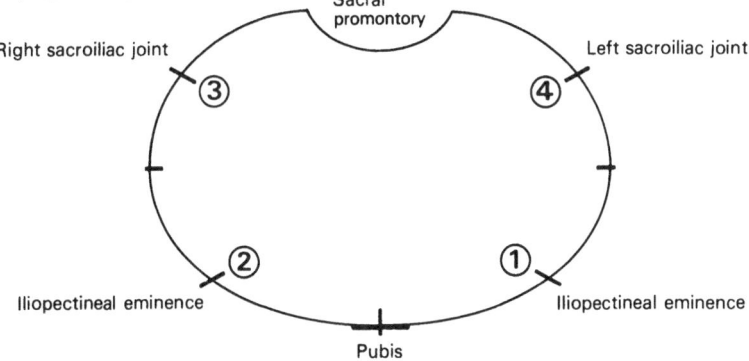

Figure 22 The pelvic inlet showing the four cardinal points used to determine fetal position

In a vertex presentation the denominator is the *occiput* and if this is entering the pelvis opposite the left iliopectineal eminence, the fetal position is described as left occipito-anterior (LOA). If the occiput is entering the pelvis opposite the right sacroiliac joint, the position is right occipito-posterior (ROP). Other examples of denominators are the *sacrum* (in breech presentations) and *mentum* (point of chin in face presentations). These matters are discussed below in Chapters 8 and 10 on mechanisms of labour and malpresentations.

The spine of the fetus is not twisted until labour is established, so its position indicates the position of the occiput; in other words, in reporting the fetal position to be LOA after abdominal palpation the practitioner has in fact felt the fetal back to be situated in the left anterior part of the uterus. The exact position of the occiput itself is determined by vaginal examination, usually during labour.

The next step in palpation is to decide whether the head (if presentation is cephalic) is *engaged* or not. 'Engaged' means that the maximum diameters have passed through the pelvic inlet, and the ability to arrive at the correct decision in this respect improves with experience. After abdominal palpation is complete, the fetal heart is checked and in most cases it is best heard over the fetal back and at a level well below the umbilicus of the woman if the head is engaged.

After the fundal height has been ascertained the lateral aspects of the uterus are palpated. Methods may vary slightly but palpation must always be gentle and movements of the hand smooth. I consider it best to palpate each side of the uterus in turn starting with the left side. By applying gentle pressure to the right side of the uterus with the entire palm of the left hand, the examiner, with the fingertips of the other hand, can identify more easily the fetal parts on the left (Figure 23). The procedure is reversed to identify the fetal parts in the right half of the uterus. The fetal back is firm and smooth, and the side in which the limbs are situated feels irregular or 'knobbly'. Limbs may move during palpation.

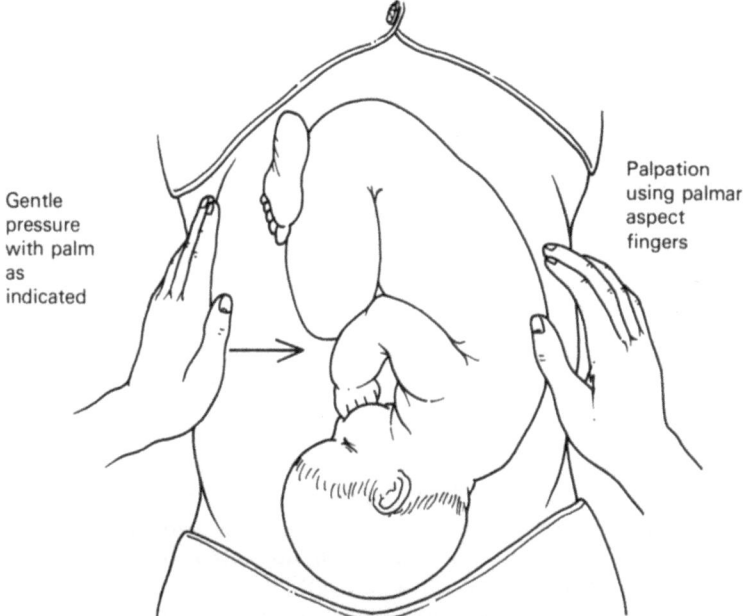

Gentle pressure with palm as indicated

Palpation using palmar aspect fingers

Figure 23   Abdominal palpation in late pregnancy

The practitioner now faces the patient's feet, and hands with fingers extended are placed on either side of the lower poles of the uterus. The head is hard and globular, and mobility may be tested by moving the fingers gently from side to side. If the head is entering the pelvis or if it is well engaged, the bony prominences are more readily felt by asking the patient to take in a deep breath, and then allowing the fingertips to slip into the pelvis as she exhales. The bony prominence of the head felt on the same side as the back is the *occiput*, and the *sinciput* is the prominence on the other side. If the head is well flexed the occipital protuberance is at a lower level in the pelvis than the brow.

The *Pawlik grip* (Figure 24) is a useful method of palpating the fetal parts entering the pelvis with the right hand which is placed suprapubically with thumb and fingers widely separated. As the patient exhales the hand is allowed to sink into the lower abdomen. This area is generally very sensitive if the head is either entering or engaged in the pelvis, so any added pressure may be painful. The 'grip', however, may be a valuable manoeuvre if properly executed. The thumb and fingertips should *not* be approximated, and the movement must be very smoothly performed.

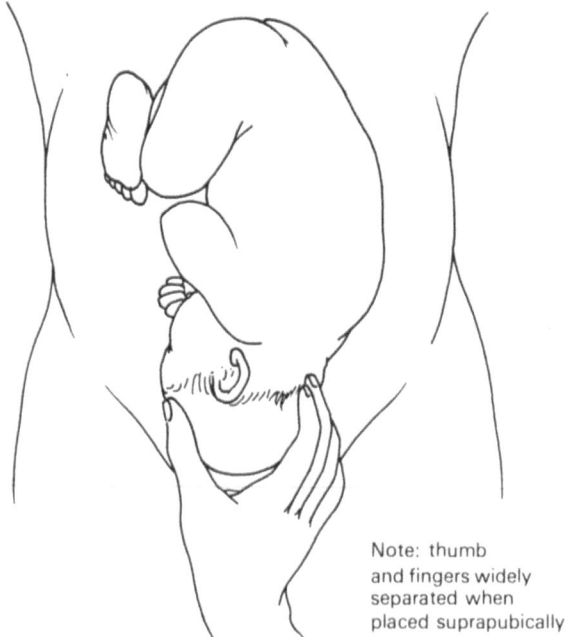

Note: thumb and fingers widely separated when placed suprapubically

Figure 24 The Pawlik grip

5

Blood testing and the anaemias of pregnancy

Blood tests performed initially in early pregnancy were mentioned in the previous chapter and haemoglobin estimations should be repeated on at least two subsequent occasions, at about 30 and 38 weeks. This is because although life-threatening anaemia is not often seen in the United Kingdom, lesser degrees of the condition are the commonest disorder found in pregnancy. In many tropical areas and developing countries, however, anaemias constitute a major cause of both maternal and perinatal mortality.

Iron-deficiency anaemia

Most cases of anaemia in the United Kingdom are associated with iron-deficiency, and as a broad generalization it may be said that women tend to be anaemic and men do not. This is so because the slight loss of iron that occurs via urine, faeces and sweat (2 mg daily) in both sexes is made good by iron absorption via the mucosa of the small intestine from a normal dietary intake. The iron loss that occurs during average menstruation, however, may amount to 30 times that lost daily by other means, and the dietary intake of iron is insufficient to compensate for this loss.

During pregnancy, the fetus and placenta make great demands on the mother's iron stores, particularly in the last trimester, and this continues throughout lactation. The increased need for iron far exceeds the saving associated with amenorrhoea.

A consideration of some physiological principles involved in the blood system during pregnancy is of value before discussing the clinical aspects. From the 12th week of pregnancy the total blood volume is increased by more than 25%, rising to between 40 and 50% in the second trimester. This change in volume is associated with the altered hormonal status in pregnancy which causes increased sodium and water retention. The increase in plasma volume, however, is greater than the increase in the volume of red blood cells, and as a result the blood is diluted, the so-called *physiological hydraemia of pregnancy*. Because of this, a simple estimation of the amount of haemoglobin in g/dl (normally about 12 to 16) may be as low as 10 without necessarily indicating iron lack. For this reason the old term physiological 'anaemia' of pregnancy was discarded and the word 'hydraemia' substituted.

However, it has been found clinically that much of the haemodilution is associated with an iron-deficiency anaemia, and even though a full blood picture and film are desirable, a haemoglobin estimation alone is of importance especially if accompanied by a haematocrit estimation.

No woman should be allowed to commence labour suffering from anaemia and treatment should be aimed at keeping the haemoglobin level above 12 g/dl (or over 80%). Anaemia increases the risks of hypotonic uterine inertia (page 177), postpartum haemorrhage and infection, and severe degrees of anaemia may be associated with an increased incidence of pre-eclampsia, prematurity and low-birthweight babies. Adequate corrective therapy with iron supplements improves the prognosis of all these conditions.

Absorbed iron is rapidly transferred to the plasma in which it is bound to a substance called *transferrin*, and in this form is conveyed to the body stores. It is released from the latter to the bone marrow as required, and it is not until these stores are exhausted that iron lack becomes evident both clinically and haematologically. As a rule a patient suffering from iron-deficient anaemia will increase her percentage absorption of ingested iron; but this is not invariably true and some patients appear not to absorb iron in pregnancy so parenteral administration is indicated. Other causes for apparent failure to respond to oral iron medication include nausea and vomiting, and some women just forget or fail to take the tablets. Less commonly there may be some hidden source of bleeding.

Megaloblastic anaemias
The importance of DNA, a component of nuclei and chromosomes, has been mentioned (page 34) and this substance is essential for cell division to occur. Folic acid and vitamin B_{12} are required for the synthesis of DNA, so the needs for these in pregnancy, when a fetus and placenta are actively growing, are greatly increased. Folic acid stores in the mother, mostly in the liver, are small and unless supplements are given deficiency is readily manifest. This will cause arrest in the development of the mature red blood cells (erythropoiesis), and the bone marrow becomes filled with megaloblasts which in severe cases may be found in the bloodstream.

FOLIC ACID DEFICIENCY

This may sometimes be seen in patients who have taken oral contraceptives for many years. Sulphonamides and anticonvulsant drugs (phenobarbitone, phenytoin, primidone) are sometimes associated with a megaloblastic anaemia. These possibilities should be borne in mind, as well as the fact that both iron and folic acid deficiency are more commonly found in twin pregnancies. Folic acid is found in iron-containing foods such as meat, liver and green vegetables, but much is destroyed by cooking.

It is possible that folic acid deficiency may play a part in abortion, abruptio placentae, prematurity and fetal abnormalities, but definite associations have not been established. Folic acid levels in the body are usually assessed by estimating the serum folate. A level below 2.0 μg/l indicates the need for immediate corrective action and additional oral supplements of 15 mg daily should be given. Symptoms of this type of anaemia, which include pallor, lassitude, dyspnoea and tachycardia, may develop rapidly.

Other anaemias

Whereas folic acid stores in the body are small, those of vitamin B_{12} are usually high, and anaemia in pregnancy due to lack of this vitamin is uncommon. *Addisonian* or pernicious anaemia associated with the absence of intrinsic factor in the stomach and failure of absorption of vitamin B_{12} is a rarity in pregnancy, as are tropical nutritional anaemias in the United Kingdom. If a patient with true Addisonian anaemia is given large doses of folic acid before the diagnosis is established, it is possible to mask the haematological picture and increase the risk of neurological complications. However, the regime described below, in which routine iron and folic acid supplements are given to almost all pregnant women, will obviate this small risk as the folic acid content is small.

Routine preventive therapy

Almost all women (the exceptions are shown below) should receive supplementary iron with small doses of folic acid during pregnancy. The aphorism 'prevention is better than cure' most certainly applies to the anaemias of pregnancy. Prophylactic treatment is delayed until after the 14th week of pregnancy to avoid possible nausea and vomiting, and oral iron may then be administered using one of the many standard preparations. The one-tablet-a-day routine is most satisfactory if available and I use tablets which contain ferrous sulphate, 160 mg with folic acid 400 g (Slow-Fe Folic) or ferrous fumarate equivalent to 100 mg of iron with folic acid 350 g (Pregaday). Acceptance and tolerance of the medication, as well as the cost and availability, are factors to consider and other proprietary preparations are used if necessary.

If response to oral medication is poor, and it is not uncommon to find the level of haemoglobin falling, intramuscular iron may be given. A course of ten injections, one every other day, of 2 ml ironsorbitol/citric acid complex (Jectofer) is administered into the buttocks.

Personally I will not prescribe undiluted iron injections for intravenous administration because unpleasant reactions may occur, including anaphylactic shock. Total dose iron infusion (using iron dextran in a saline drip containing heparin) may be considered in rare cases where blood transfusion is not permitted. If blood transfusion is needed to ensure that a patient does not commence labour in a grossly anaemic state, it is often preferable to give packed cells very slowly as there is the risk of overloading the circulatory system in view of the physiological hydraemia present.

The haemoglobinopathies

Haemoglobin (Hb), a pigment found in the red blood cells of animals, exists in many varieties. Each animal species has a different form, and in humans the adult form HbA differs from that of the fetus HbF. The haemoglobin molecule consists of the iron-containing, oxygen carrying 'haem' group plus 'globin' portion, and numerous abnormal types of haemoglobin are known. Haemoglobinopathies are forms of genetically inherited haemolytic anaemias. Some people may have the majority of their haemoglobin in an abnormal form if the appropriate gene has been inherited from both parents (homozygous), while others with the condition in its heterozygous form may have mostly the normal HbA in their erythrocytes. The two most common conditions seen are thalassaemia and sickle-cell anaemia.

THALASSAEMIA
This is found in peoples inhabiting parts of South East Asia and the Mediterranean littoral, including Greece, Turkey, Italy and Cyprus. The defect causes destruction of immature erythrocytes, a process which is accelerated in pregnancy when severe anaemia may develop rapidly. In the homozygous patient (*Cooley's anaemia*) early death is reported from infection or heart failure and pregnancy is rarely seen. The condition is much less severe in its heterozygous form (*thalassaemia minor*). Although there is a chronic haemolytic anaemia due to the destruction of the fragile red cells, serum iron is normal or raised,

and marked bone marrow activity leads to a depletion of folic acid stores.

Treatment

Iron therapy is contraindicated, but folic acid, 10 to 20 mg daily, is given. Blood transfusions, which may depress erythropoiesis, may be needed in a haemolytic crisis.

SICKLE-CELL ANAEMIA

The most frequent abnormal haemoglobin found in this condition is HbS, and it occurs in some black races. The normal erythrocyte lives for 100 to 120 days, but those containing abnormal haemoglobins may survive for 1 or 2 weeks only. Haemolytic crises may occur with rapidity, especially in late pregnancy, and are accompanied by exacerbation of anaemia, jaundice and pyrexia. When the oxygen content of the erythrocyte is reduced, the cell becomes sickle-shaped, as reduced HbS is far less soluble than oxy-HbS and crystallizes out of solution. The resultant 'sludging' increases blood viscosity, and intracapillary thromboses may affect bones, spleen, gut and kidneys causing severe pain. In addition to hypoxia, acidosis and trauma may precipitate a painful or 'sludging' crisis while infection can lead to a 'haemolytic' crisis.

In most heterozygous patients, the amount of HbS present is less than that of normal HbA and few problems arise during pregnancy and labour, provided there is no hypoxia. Anaesthesia today should cause no problem when administered by properly equipped skilled personnel.

Treatment

This is as for thalassaemia – folic acid but not iron is given. Blood transfusion carries considerable risk in sickle-cell disease and may precipitate aplastic anaemia. Infections require immediate treatment with the appropriate antibiotic, acidosis is avoided by oral sodium bicarbonate administration, and heparin is given if thromboses and infarction occur.

6

Urine analysis and its significance

The advent of plastic strips that can be dipped into urine to detect the presence of protein, glucose, acetone and other abnormal constituents has considerably eased the task of those supervising prenatal care in some parts of the world. It is, of course, mandatory to test urine at every routine examination of the pregnant woman. The strips are useful for screening purposes, although with some a good eye for colour and the means for accurate timing are required! In other areas the older practice of boiling the upper half of a tube of urine to detect protein may still be necessary, and Fehling's and Benedict's solutions are used to diagnose glycosuria. The importance in prenatal care lies more in ensuring that urine is examined satisfactorily than in the methods employed.

Abnormal constituents most commonly found in urine are protein (proteinuria) glucose (glycosuria) and acetone (ketonuria), and all may have a significance that must not be ignored.

Proteinuria
The most important causes of proteinuria in pregnancy are:

(1)   Pre-eclampsia.
(2)   Contamination of the specimen.
(3)   Urinary tract infection.
(4)   Chronic renal disease.
(5)   Postural or orthostatic albuminuria.
(6)   General diseases, for example, congestive cardiac failure and some acute specific fevers.

PRE-ECLAMPSIA
Although listed first pre-eclampsia is not the commonest cause of proteinuria in the United Kingdom. It is, however, of major importance and is discussed separately in Chapter 14.

CONTAMINATION OF THE SPECIMEN
Contamination may be associated with an infective vaginal discharge, blood or liquor, or the contaminant may be present in the receptacle in which the specimen is collected. To eliminate these causes, the vulva should be swabbed with cotton wool dipped in sterile water and a clean midstream specimen of urine (MSU) received into a sterile container. Suprapubic aspiration or catheterization of the bladder should not be necessary.

URINARY TRACT INFECTION
Urological disorders must not be dismissed as simple urinary tract infections, as they may be associated with structural abnormalities of the kidney or lead to involvement of the renal parenchyma and chronic renal disease. Thus repeated attacks of cystitis or haematuria indicate the need for full urinary tract investigation. When the patient is pregnant and intravenous pyelography, for example, cannot be performed, such investigations may be delayed until after the post-natal examination. However, any urinary infection must be identified, treated and eradicated. A condition once diagnosed as acute pyelitis of pregnancy should more correctly be called acute pyelonephritis, a term which clearly shows the inherent risk of chronic renal disease. Clinical features of the condition include pyrexia, vomiting, rigors and loin tenderness, with urgency and frequency of micturition and dysuria due to the accompanying cystitis. Many published accounts report that about 30% of women who undergo full follow-up investigation after acute urinary tract infection show radiological abnormalities in the renal tract.

Bacteria may be found in a specimen of freshly voided urine passed by a woman displaying no signs or symptoms of infection. This is known as *asymptomatic bacteriuria* and where possible a bacteria count should be performed routinely at the first prenatal examination. A count of 100 000 per ml or more is significant and indicates that bacteria are multiplying in the urinary tract. Over 25% of women with significant asymptomatic bacteriuria develop pyelonephritis unless active treatment is given. Organisms may reach the kidney by ascending infection from the vulva via the urethra, bladder and ureter. The tendency for this to occur in pregnancy is increased because:

(1)   Vesico-ureteric reflux (that is, urine passes from bladder to ureter) associated with a lax sphincter occurs.
(2)   The ureters (especially the right) may be compressed by the gravid uterus.
(3)   Although the ureteric muscle hypertrophies, the degree of hypertrophy may be inadequate to overcome the dilatation, kink-

ing, and diminished peristaltic activity that is found in the ureters in pregnancy (the latter are possibly progesterone effects).

As a result of these factors, urinary tract stasis occurs. Catheterization of the bladder, coitus and dysuria (the last is seen quite commonly in the immediate postpartum period) all tend to increase the risk of ascending infection.

Thus when a patient who is symptom-free and has no previous history of urinary infection is found to have a bacteriuria count of 100 000 or more, the test should be repeated; if there is still evidence of significant asymptomatic bacteriuria, the responsible organism (often *Escherichia coli*) should be identified and treatment prescribed. After treatment, urine specimens should be cultured fortnightly to ensure that infection has been eradicated.

Treatment

Various modes of treatment may be considered, and these include ampicillin 250 mg, nitrofurantoin (Furadantin) 100 mg, or nalidixic acid (Negram) 1 g − all three drugs are given 6-hourly for 8 days. Sulphonamides should not be prescribed in the last 6 weeks of pregnancy or during lactation as they cross the placental barrier, are excreted in milk, and can lead to jaundice in the newborn. In fact I prefer to avoid sulphonamides in pregnancy at any stage and have effectively utilized intermittent ampicillin therapy to prevent relapses of infection, the patient taking the medication for 1 week in 4. Cephalosporins are used occasionally but one cannot overstress the importance of avoiding all medication during pregnancy − particularly during the first 4 months − unless definite indications exist.

The list above is not intended to include all forms of therapy in use, but special mention must be given to an old hospital standby 'Mist. Pot. Cit. et Soda Bic.' usually a most unpleasant-tasting mixture but an effective remedy to combat *E. coli* urinary infection. The organism thrives in acid urine, so the mixture must thus be given in adequate quantities to ensure that every specimen or urine passed is alkaline. Tetracyclines and sulphamethoxazole-trimethoprim (Septrin) are contraindicated in pregnancy.

CHRONIC KIDNEY DISEASE

The care of pregnant women suffering from chronic kidney disease is generally in the hands of consultants from diverse disciplines, and ideally the patient would be best cared for in hospitals with specialized renal units. It is essential, however, to be aware of some aspects of this subject. Analgesic nephropathy (phenacetin) with associated papillary necrosis, polycystic kidney disease, renal tuberculosis and nephropathy associated with systemic (disseminated) lupus erythematosus (SLE) are rare complications of pregnancy. The nephrotic syndrome which is associated with marked oedema and albuminuria and usually normal renal function is also rare.

The most common form of chronic renal disease seen in pregnancy in the United Kingdom is chronic pyelonephritis, and here prognosis must be guarded as a patient with this condition is more likely to develop a superimposed pre-eclampsia. If renal function is normal and hypertension not severe mother and baby should do well. If, however, renal function is impaired, and especially in the presence of retinal changes, prognosis is poor.

The following points are helpful in establishing the diagnosis:

(1)   The patient's history (for example, a previous history of acute pyelonephritis).
(2)   The urine, in addition to protein, will contain granular and cellular casts and possibly red and white blood cells from the onset of pregnancy.
(3)   Iron-deficiency anaemia may accompany chronic pyelonephritis.
(4)   Renal biopsy may be performed.
(5)   A high titre of agglutinating antibodies to *E. coli* will suggest renal tissue infection.

Impairment of renal function may be shown by:

(1)   A raised serum creatinine. Creatinine clearance is used as a measure of the glomerular filtration rate and this is considerably increased in normal pregnancy thereby lowering the serum level of this substance.
(2)   Raised levels of urea or urea nitrogen in whole blood or serum. The whole blood level is approximately 10% below plasma level and approximately 50% of urea is urea nitrogen.
(3)   Inability to concentrate urine above a specific gravity of 1.020.

ORTHOSTATIC OR POSTURAL ALBUMINURIA
In pregnancy this is due to renal congestion associated with hypertrophy of the renal arteries and pressure on the veins by the enlarging uterus. The lumbar lordosis of pregnancy tends to increase the pressure effects. Proteinuria is found in the one specimen of urine passed after a change of posture, for example, the first specimen on rising from bed. To diagnose the condition the patient may be observed in hospital for 48 hours and all specimens passed are tested. Diagnosis is confirmed if only one specimen per day contains protein. The condition is of no significance.

Glycosuria

An isolated finding of glucose in the urine during pregnancy is by no means uncommon and in most cases is of no significance. Diabetes in pregnancy, however, is associated with a high perinatal mortality and the patient requires the closest supervision by the obstetrician and physician with a special interest in the condition. The cause or type of glycosuria is determined by the glucose tolerance test, the results of which are best interpreted by plotting the findings on a graph. When a glucose tolerance test is performed the patient fasts overnight (for at least 12 hours), and thereafter a fasting blood sample for glucose estimation is taken and urine tested. The patient is then given 50 g of glucose dissolved in 300 ml water to drink within a time limit of 5 minutes. Blood sugar estimations are made every half hour and, if produced, a specimen of urine is tested at the same time. Minimal urine testing requires examination of specimens at 60 and 120 minutes so tests will take at least 2 hours to complete.

To interpret the results it is essential to understand the term *renal threshold*. Glucose is a threshold substance which means that the renal tubular cells have a limited capacity to reabsorb it. The normal renal threshold for glucose is 10 mmol/l (180 mg/100 ml). So when the concentration of glucose in the bloodstream is below this level, all the glucose in the glomerular filtrate is reabsorbed and none appears in the urine. If the threshold is exceeded, there is glycosuria.

The normal glucose tolerance test curve is shown in Figure 25. The salient features are:

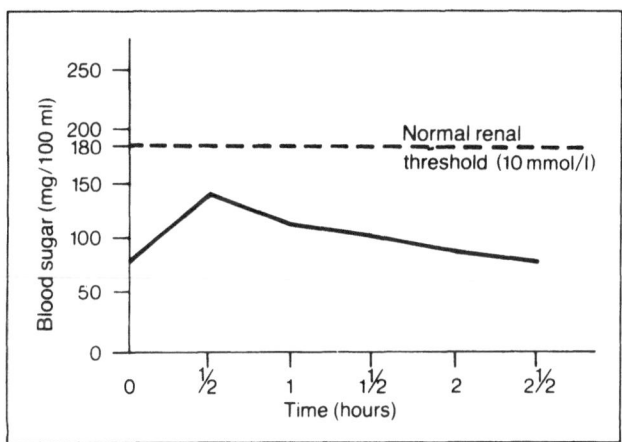

Figure 25   The normal glucose tolerance test curve

(1)   The fasting blood glucose level does not exceed 5.55 mmol/l (100 mg/100 ml).
(2)   The curve rises quickly after the glucose meal but the blood sugar concentration never exceeds the normal renal threshold.
(3)   Within 2 to 2½ hours blood sugar level has returned almost to the fasting level. The diminution in blood sugar is slower than in the non-pregnant state because of increased levels of oestrogen, progesterone and placental lactogen.
(4)   At no time is there glycosuria.

Glycosuria in pregnancy may be either renal or alimentary glycosuria, or associated with diabetes mellitus.

RENAL GLYCOSURIA
Renal glycosuria occurs because there is a lowering of the normal renal threshold, which may fall even to below 5.55 mmol/l (100 mg/100 ml). The lowering of renal threshold is due to the increased glomerular filtration that occurs in pregnancy making the tubules unable to reabsorb the additional amounts of glucose presented to them. Renal glycosuria is not uncommon, occurs in the second half of pregnancy and disappears after delivery. The glucose tolerance curve is as the normal curve but some of the urine specimens show the presence of glycosuria. The condition is believed to be of no significance.

ALIMENTARY GLYCOSURIA
The old term for the graph which leads to the diagnosis of alimentary glycosuria (Figure 26) is the 'lag curve' and this is most descriptive. The term was used because although insulin secretion is normal, the hormonal changes in pregnancy make the insulin response sluggish or cause it to 'lag' behind. Thus after a 50 g glucose meal the blood sugar level rises rapidly to above the renal threshold, but then a normal flow of insulin causes a rapid fall, and blood sugar level is generally below its fasting value within 1 to 2 hours. The specimen of urine passed after the blood glucose level rises above 10 mmol/l (180 mg/100 ml) will show glycosuria.

The explanation given above for alimentary glycosuria affords an easy method of visualizing the cause for the condition, although it is too simplistic as control of glucose metabolism is complex. In addition to insulin produced by the beta-cells of the pancreatic islets of Langerhans, many other hormones are involved (glucagon, made in the alpha-cells of the islets of Langerhans, and the anterior pituitary growth hormone both raise blood sugar levels, and adrenal and placental hormones also affect carbohydrate metabolism). Some associate the condition with a rapid emptying of the stomach in pregnancy so that

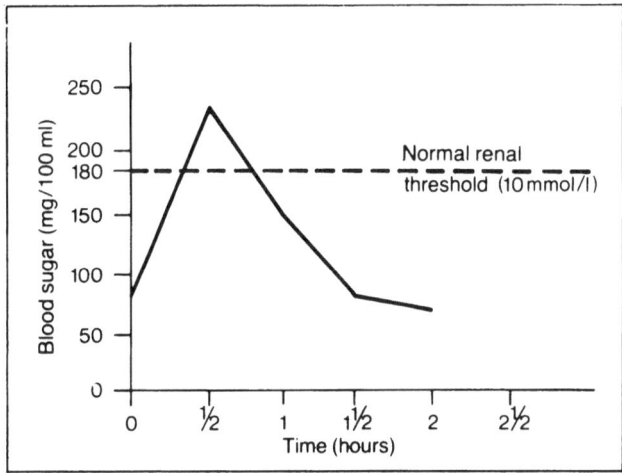

Figure 26 Alimentary glycosuria – the 'lag' curve

glucose is absorbed very quickly from the intestine. Alimentary glycosuria is quite common in early pregnancy and is of no significance.

Prior to a consideration of aspects of diabetes in pregnancy it may
be noted that there is a *'flat' glucose tolerance test curve* in which
the blood sugar level rises slowly and by less than 2.8 mmol/1
(50 mg/100 ml) after a glucose meal. It is found in normal healthy
individuals and is not uncommon in pregnancy; the fasting blood
sugar level is normal. It is probably associated with malabsorption of
glucose and, although rarely it may be due to lack of growth hormone
or adrenal glucocorticoids, it is generally of no significance and glycosuria is not a feature.

DIABETES MELLITUS
The features of the glucose tolerance curve in diabetes mellitus (Figure
27) are:

(1)   High fasting blood sugar (6 mmol/1 (110 mg/100 ml)) or more
is diagnostic).
(2)   A curve rising rapidly to above the renal threshold.
(3)   The blood sugar level remaining well above its fasting value
after 2 or even 3 hours.

Latent diabetes may be unmasked by pregnancy. The fasting blood
sugar is normal, the peak rises above the normal renal threshold of
10 mmol/1 (180 mg/100 ml) and after 2 hours is more than 6.7 mmol/1
(120 mg/100 ml).

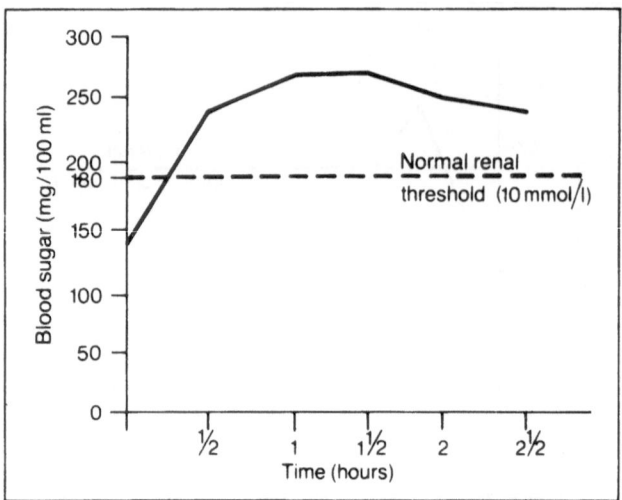

Figure 27   The diabetic glucose tolerance test curve

DIABETES IN PREGNANCY

Before the discovery of insulin by Banting and Best in 1922 diabetes was associated with hypoplasia of the genital tract. Diabetic women tended to have amenorrhoea or scanty, infrequent periods and were often subfertile, probably fortunately as pregnancy in diabetics in the pre-insulin era was associated with a perinatal mortality of over 50%, and many of the women sufferers were dead within 2 years.

Insulin changed this picture completely and today the controlled diabetic is no less fertile than her non-diabetic counterpart. Maternal risk is increased, but only slightly provided that there is constant specialist care. Maternal mortality in the United Kingdom is still below 0.5% although, for example, the incidence of pre-eclampsia with its attendant complications is higher and the necessity for caesarean section is more common. Perinatal mortality, too, has fallen very considerably and although the overall figure remains at approximately 10% or more, specialized centres have reduced this figure to below 3%. However, if diabetic complications such as retinopathy, nephropathy or vascular disease are present, risks to both mother and baby are much increased.

Management

The physician supervises the control of the disease, and except in the most minor cases where special dietary measures may suffice, insulin (soluble and possible the isophane variety) is administered. Since, for reasons already specified, other causes for glycosuria are common in pregnancy, insulin requirements cannot be judged purely on urine examinations and regular blood sugar estimations are necessary. Admission to hospital for stabilization in early pregnancy and again late in the mid-trimester when insulin requirements often increase, may be indicated. Most patients will require admission when 32 to 34 weeks pregnant for rest, observation and frequent blood examination to ensure good stabilization of the disorder and to avoid hypoglycaemia and ketosis.

Maternal complications
Three important complications of diabetes in pregnancy are:

(1) *Candidal (monilial) vaginitis.* This fungus is one of the few common vaginal infecting organisms that thrives in an acid environment and in pregnancy the pH of the vagina may fall to below 4. Glycosuria predisposes to the growth of candida, and pregnant diabetic patients are prone to this form of vaginitis. The associated pruritus is often intense and causes the patient considerable distress. Various modes of treatment include:

(a) Nystatin pessaries intravaginally, one per night for 15 nights.
(b) Clotrimazole vaginal tablets (Canesten) one per night for 6 days, or two per night for 3 days.
(c) Painting the vagina with 1% aqueous solution of gentian violet on six occasions over 2 weeks, an old form of treatment which is quite effective and still in use. The disadvantages of the therapy include the difficulty in keeping the dye localized solely to the vagina. However, a considerable advantage is gained by mopping out the vagina with pledgets of cotton wool moistened in 1% sodium bicarbonate to precede the course of paintings. This can give instant relief by removing much of the fungus.
(d) Miconazole cream or pessaries intravaginally, one per night for 1 week.

(2) Pre-eclampsia.
(3) Hydramnios.

Pre-eclampsia and hydramnios may well be manifest in the last weeks of pregnancy and indicate the essential need for rest and observation in hospital.

Any infection may upset carbohydrate balance and must be avoided where possible. Patients should be advised to keep away from overcrowded places. If infection occurs, the causative organism must be identified and appropriate treatment instituted, after ensuring that the antibiotic or any other drug considered essential is safe for use in pregnancy (the *Data Sheet Compendium* issued to all doctors in the United Kingdom is invaluable). Diabetic patients should have urine specimens examined routinely and bacterial counts performed, and asymptomatic bacteriuria should be treated (page 63).

The newborn baby of the diabetic mother is usually large, oedematous and lethargic. It is more likely to suffer from respiratory distress syndrome or hyaline membrane disease and to develop respiratory and metabolic acidosis, hyperkalaemia and hypoglycaemia. The dysmature infant is best cared for in an intensive neonatal care unit with monitoring of blood gases, pH values and blood sugar.

Termination of pregnancy

Since complications occur so frequently in the latter weeks of pregnancy, perinatal mortality is greatly reduced by preterm delivery. Although there can be no hard and fast rules in obstetric judgement, pregnancies are often terminated at about 37 weeks. Monitoring of placental efficiency, ultrasonic scanning of uterus and baby, and amniocentesis for lecithin–sphingomyelin (or LS) ratio (see page 191) aid the obstetrician in deciding when to recommend delivery. Surgical induction of labour with oxytocic infusion may be carried out or, if conditions for this are unfavourable, caesarean section may be preferred.

Insulin requirements for the patient generally decrease in the immediate days postpartum, as placental hormones are no longer present. Dosage may vary widely at this time and depend upon blood and urine examinations. To obtain the best results for mothers and babies in diabetes, care by specialized teams is an advantage.

The prediabetic state

About 30 years ago, it was noted that women who subsequently developed diabetes gave birth to very large babies and that pregnancy was associated with a high perinatal mortality. The nature of this prediabetic state is unknown, although overaction of the anterior pituitary has been suggested as a possible mechanism. The patient shows no clinical evidence of the disorder and the glucose tolerance test is normal and may remain so for many years. Women who give birth to large babies (4.5 kg (10 lb) or over) may well be in the prediabetic state and this condition should be considered especially if the patient is adipose, has a family history of the disorder or develops pre-eclampsia or hydramnios.

Large babies may, however, be a normal feature in some healthy families and these infants are usually active and give no undue cause for concern in their first days of life. Large babies associated with a maternal prediabetic state, however, are lethargic and require the same intensive care as babies born to mothers with clinical diabetes. Although the glucose tolerance test is normal, it is possible that a repeat test after giving the patient cortisone may produce a curve showing some of the features found in diabetics.

SUGGESTED ROUTINE WHEN GLYCOSURIA IS FOUND
It has been shown that glycosuria in pregnancy is found quite commonly and in the majority of cases it is unnecessary to give the patient cause for concern by requesting full glucose tolerance tests. Urine should be tested for glucose at every prenatal visit and, if found on more than one occasion, a random blood sugar estimation is indicated. This may be performed 1 to 2 hours after breakfast or lunch or may be a fasting specimen. If the blood sugar level is below 5 mmol/l (90 mg/100 ml), the patient is not a diabetic. However, if there is any doubt at all a full glucose tolerance test should be performed.

Ketonuria
In the diabetic patient, ketosis is particularly dangerous to the fetus and must be avoided by correct management of the disorder. Ketone bodies may be found in the urine in association with vomiting due to any cause or with an inadequate diet.

In labour, especially when prolonged, dehydration and ketosis must be corrected. Muscle cells in these conditions become depleted of potassium, and hypotonic uterine inertia and postpartum haemorrhage are more likely. Intravenous 10% glucose may be administered.

7

The physiology of labour

Labour is the process by which the fetus and the placenta and membranes are expelled through the birth canal. The three stages are:

(1)   The first stage − from the onset of labour to full dilatation of the cervix.
(2)   The second stage − from full dilatation of the cervix to the delivery of the baby.
(3)   The third stage − from the delivery of the baby to the delivery of the placenta and membranes.

Although the duration of the second and third stages may be assessed with accuracy, it is more difficult to estimate the duration of the first stage as the timing of onset is not clearly defined. Yet it is important for the expectant mother to be confident of knowing when labour has started so that she may seek skilled assistance. The importance of confidence, knowledge, parentcraft classes and relaxation exercises has been discussed in Chapter 4 on prenatal care, and as term approaches the patient should be told that she should not hesitate to contact her midwife or doctor if she believes that labour has started.
The onset of labour is indicated by:

(1)   the occurrence of painful contractions occurring with regularity;
(2)   a 'show' of blood-stained mucus; or less commonly
(3)   the 'breaking of the waters' (that is, a vaginal loss of amniotic fluid).

During her pregnancy the patient should learn that it is common for expectant mothers to complain of a low backache which increases slightly as term approaches and the head engages. The pressure feeling associated with this should not, however, cause undue inconvenience. The mother is informed that when labour starts the discomfort spreads to the lower abdomen, and that labour is considered to be established (or the first stage has commenced) when regular uterine contractions occur every 10 minutes or more frequently.

What the 'show' is and why it occurs, and the timing and significance of the rupture of the membranes are discussed below, but one cannot overstress the importance of ensuring that the women whose pregnancy is nearing its end knows she has the continuous support of her attendants.

Prolonged labour can be disastrous to both mother and baby – the old definition of this was a labour which lasted 48 hours or more. This should be very rare indeed today, yet women not uncommonly notice a 'show' a day or more before regular contractions occur. Premature rupture of the membranes may occur long before term and is not without risk. The timing of the onset of the first stage of labour thus depends upon the patient's own story and the practitioner's observations. When painful uterine contractions are occurring regularly, and are associated with a cervix that is effacing and dilated by 3 cm or more, the patient is in established, active labour.

The onset of labour
The causes of the spontaneous onset of labour remain obscure but without doubt a variety of factors is involved. The onset of labour is marked physiologically by the commencement of *retraction* which is a phenomenon unique to uterine muscle in labour and which results in permanent shortening of the fibres.

Most of the growth of the uterus in pregnancy is due to proliferation of the myometrium with muscle cells increasing both in size and number. The muscle fibres of the uterus in late pregnancy and in labour are arranged in three indefinite overlapping layers:

(1) Outer longitudinal fibres which form a relatively thin layer.
(2) A thick mass of middle interlacing fibres which run spirally downwards and inwards to form an interdigitating network perforated by the spiral arterioles and vessels supplying the decidua and placenta.
(3) Inner circular fibres (see Figure 51, page 176).

The musculature is most abundant in the upper uterine segment and the fibres thin out as they approach the cervix. Thus, in normal labour the upper segment is actively contracting and retracting, while the lower segment is more elastic and relatively passive. Contractions, in which muscle fibres shorten but then regain fully their original length, may be appreciated by palpation in the latter weeks of pregnancy

(Braxton—Hicks painless contractions). The precise mechanism that triggers off labour and causes regular contractions with retraction, and of which the patient is aware (the 'pains'), is unknown.

The biochemistry of muscle activity is most complex, and difficulty in determining the cause of the onset of labour is increased because the innervation of the uterus is not fully understood. The uterine muscle is supplied by the autonomic nervous system but evidence as regards the relative activity of the sympathetic and parasympathetic systems is conflicting. Alpha (α) and beta (β) receptor sites in the muscle have been described, the former exciting and the latter inhibiting activity. Thus, as an example of practical application of this knowledge, beta-adrenergic stimulants such as salbutamol are sometimes used to inhibit uterine activity in preterm labour. Hormones may well affect or even control the activity of these sites.

That preterm labour is not uncommon in twin pregnancies or in association with hydramnios suggests that mechanical stimulation may play a part in determining the onset of labour. However, labour is often induced by forewater rupture (amniotomy) which diminishes uterine volume and thus muscular stretching, although aspiration of fluid via the abdominal wall (amniocentesis) does not have this effect. Other factors are thus exercising an influence here, and again these are probably hormonal.

It would appear, therefore, that hormones play the most important role in regulating uterine activity. In late pregnancy the level of plasma oestradiol rises while that of progesterone (possibly an inhibitor of uterine activity) falls. Oestrogens may stimulate the decidual cells to release *prostaglandins* which have a powerful stimulating or oxytocic effect on uterine contractions. Oxytocin secreted by the posterior pituitary gland and by the fetus itself may play a part in initiating labour.

Physiology of the first stage
The first stage of labour is concerned with the dilatation and 'taking-up' of the cervix and isthmus of the uterus (that is, the lower segment) and the sequence of events is as follows:

(1)   Waves of contraction and retraction begin in the area of the cornua, and as they pass downwards become less intense as the fibres thin out, so that the lower pole of the uterus is passive.
(2)   The retraction or permanent shortening of the muscles leads to an increase in intrauterine pressure which causes (3) below.
(3)   The membranes herniate into the cervical canal which dilates

slightly. This expels the mucus plug (of secretion and desquamated cells) which is stained with blood as capillary bleeding occurs when the membranes are detached from the uterine wall. This is the '*show*'.

The flexed head in the pelvis acts as a ball-valve thereby dividing the amniotic fluid in which the fetus lies into the forewaters and hind-waters. The bag of forewaters, usually very small, is well protected and thus normally does not rupture early in labour although the strength of the membranes shows considerable individual variation. In fact, in perfect normal labour the forewaters should remain intact until the second stage commences.

The longitudinal and interlacing muscle fibres spiralling downwards from the body of the uterus to the cervix exert a pulling-up action as they retract, and the internal os opens first as the lower segment thins and dilates. Effacement usually occurs early in labour in primigravidae, but often after some degree of cervical dilatation in multiparae.

As the first stage progresses the upper segment becomes thicker and the lower segment thins and is taken up. Where thick meets thin (in other words where the two segments meet) the physiological *retraction ring* is formed. In obstructed labour (Chapter 19) a pathological retraction ring or ring of Bandl is of considerable clinical significance.

Physiology of the second stage
At about the time the cervix becomes fully dilated, in the ideal normal labour the forewaters rupture. Before this, the forces acting on the fetal sac are distributed equally around the entire area. When the fore-waters rupture, a uterine contraction results in driving the fetus down-wards. A simple analogy to help in understanding this may be made by picturing the fetal sac as a balloon filled with water. Provided the skin of the balloon remains intact, pressure applied anywhere will be distributed equally around its surface. If, however, the balloon is pricked with a pin and then squeezed, the increased pressure inside it will be transmitted totally to the minute hole from which the water will spurt with some force. The pinprick can be compared to the ruptured fore-waters (Figure 28).

The fetus being pushed in a downwards direction meets considerable resistance from the soft parts especially the pelvic floor and vagina. Advance is maintained by an increase in uterine retraction. When the head stretches the pelvic floor a reflex action causes *bearing down* in which the diaphragm is fixed at the height of an inspiration and the patient's abdominal muscles contract. The practitioner is aware that the second stage has been reached as the patient cannot

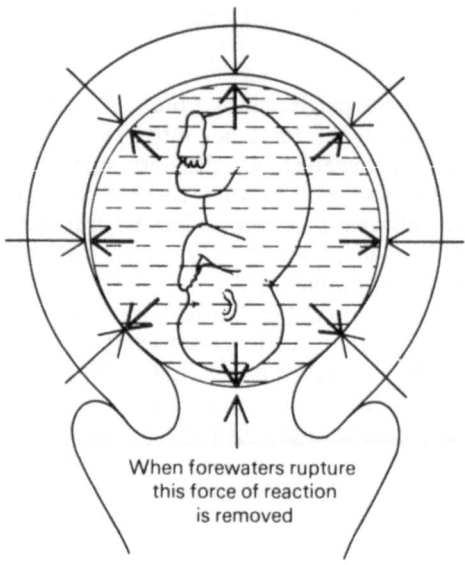

Figure 28   Physiology of the second stage of labour

stop straining down unless she pants in and out with the mouth open.
The 'bearing down' to deliver the baby may be augmented by conscious maternal effort but often this is unnecessary.

Physiology of the third stage
After the baby is born retraction of the myometrium is rapid and so
marked that the placental site is diminished to about half its original
area. The cotyledons of the placenta bunch up especially in the central
area which is torn away from the underlying decidual wall. The plane
of separation is through the deep spongy layer of the decidua basalis.
Retroplacental bleeding occurs and further contraction and retraction
forces the blood peripherally so that the entire placenta separates and
descends into the vagina. When this has occurred and the uterine
cavity is completely empty, haemorrhage from torn decidual blood
vessels will cease as the interlacing muscle fibres contract upon them in
a way often described as 'living ligatures'. Full contraction and
retraction of the myometrium when the uterine cavity is empty requires
a normal muscular tone.
   The management of the third stage of labour and of postpartum
haemorrhage is of fundamental importance in obstetrics.

Postpartum haemorrhage and the management of the third stage of labour
Postpartum haemorrhage is diagnosed when there is a vaginal loss of 500 ml or more of blood after the delivery of the baby and up to the end of the puerperium (6 weeks). A smaller loss can also be called postpartum haemorrhage, if accompanied by deterioration in the mother's physical condition, but there are causes of postpartum shock other than haemorrhage. Furthermore, blood loss after delivery cannot be measured precisely even if stained pads and swabs, etc. are weighed before and after the baby is born. The tendency to under-estimate the total blood loss is to be avoided.

Postpartum haemorrhage may be divided into primary, which occurs within 24 hours of delivery, and secondary, which occurs subsequently during the puerperium.

CAUSES OF POSTPARTUM HAEMORRHAGE
Traumatic
Bleeding from a lacerated cervix, vagina or perineum may be considerable and will continue even though the uterus is empty and well retracted. Treatment of necessity includes visualization of the bleeding area and suturing to achieve haemostasis and repair of torn tissues.

From the placental site
More commonly, however, haemorrhage occurs from the placental site. This means that part of the placenta has separated through the spongy layer of the decidua (there would be no loss from torn maternal vessels if no separation had occurred) and the myometrium has not contracted and retracted fully to occlude the blood vessels.

The causes of *incomplete retraction* are

(1)   The uterine cavity is not empty. This may be due to retained placenta and/or membranes, or blood clot.
(2)   Poor uterine muscle tone may be present. A hypotonic myometrium may be due to

(a)   Prolonged labour.
(b)   Overdistension of the uterus, which may be associated with multiple pregnancy, hydramnios or a very large baby.
(c)   Grand multiparity. The woman who has previously had four or more pregnancies is at a greater risk of several obstetric complications including postpartum haemorrhage.
(d)   Fibroids may interfere with muscular action.
(e)   A debilitated or anaemic patient. The importance of treating antepartum anaemia has been stressed and it should be

remembered that a patient who has sustained a severe antepartum haemorrhage has a greater risk of postpartum
haemorrhage.
(f)   Prolonged general anaesthesia – a rare cause today.
(g)   Hormonal causes. This is a most important group and in
      practical terms it means that there is no immediately appar-
      ent cause for failure of the uterus to retract fully. There
      may be a deficiency of prostaglandin or posterior pituitary
      oxytocin or possibly there is some intrinsic defect in the
      muscle itself (at the receptor sites mentioned earlier).

The causes of retained placenta

Hypotonic uterine action. These are listed above under (a) to (g). An
important additional cause is a *full bladder* which may inhibit proper
myometrial activity. A woman must not be allowed to commence the
second stage of labour with a distended bladder. Normally catheterization is to be avoided where possible and especially for urine testing
when a clean midstream specimen may be adequate. In labour, however, a full bladder can cause delay in all stages and catheterization is
often necessary.

Adhesions. Morbid adhesions of the placenta may be present
with no obvious cause. Overzealous curettage may possibly be a
factor in some cases where damage has been inflicted on the underlying myometrium. In the condition of *placenta accreta* the spongy
layer of the decidua has not been differentiated. The condition is rare,
and if complete there should be no placental separation and thus no
bleeding. In the past, maternal deaths occurred when the obstetrician
attempted manual removal and, unable to identify the usually obvious
plane of separation, attempted piecemeal removal of the placenta. The
condition, if not associated with haemorrhage, is best dealt with
by cutting the cord as high in the birth canal as possible and leaving
the placenta to absorb *in situ*. The patient will require antibiotic cover
as there is a high risk of infection. Many women have become pregnant after this conservative treatment, and hysterectomy, recommended for the condition in the past, may thus be avoided.

'Hour glass' contraction ring. Spasm of circular muscle fibres may
cause a contraction (or constriction) ring above which the partially or
wholly separated placenta is trapped. The term 'hour glass' is most apt
as the ring which is felt on internal examination may be so tight that it
will not even admit one finger (Figure 29). The causes of this marked
irritability of the muscle include injudicious manipulation of the
uterus during the management of the third stage and the unwise use of
oxytocic drugs. Contraction rings sometimes occur without obvious
cause and may be associated with intrinsic hormonal imbalance.

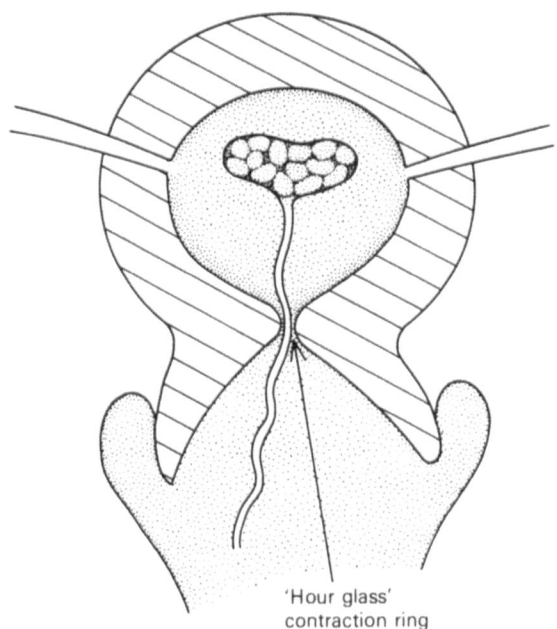

'Hour glass'
contraction ring

Figure 29   Hour glass contraction ring

MANAGEMENT OF THE THIRD STAGE OF LABOUR
Postpartum haemorrhage may often be avoided by correct management of the third stage of labour, and this is either usually in the hands
of the practitioner. Methods taught may vary as there are two normal
ways of completing this stage of labour. The patient must be under
continuous observation and in the absence of untoward haemorrhage
there is no necessity for haste. The placenta and membranes usually
separate and descend within minutes, especially if an oxytocic drug has
been injected during the baby's delivery (page 84).

Many authorities recommend that the midwife waits for the signs of
separation and descent to be manifest before completing this stage of
labour; these signs are:

(1)   The cord protruding from the vulva lengthens and this is
accompanied by a spurt of blood.
(2)   The uterine fundus rises in the abdomen usually to above the
level of the umbilicus and becomes very hard, spherical and mobile
(not unlike a cricket ball). This is due to the empty uterus being displaced upwards by the descent of the placenta into the vagina.
(3)   Gentle suprapubic pressure raising the uterus higher into the

abdomen will not be accompanied by a corresponding movement of the cord. This manoeuvre is often unnecessary.

(4) If the placenta is in the vagina it may be felt on vaginal examination. This examination, too, should rarely be necessary and increases the risk of introducing infection.

However, it is not essential to wait for complete separation and descent if the placenta is to be delivered by controlled cord traction provided the latter is applied only if and when the uterus is in a state of contraction. (The word 'controlled' often used is unnecessary as all actions in midwifery are controlled). The left hand placed suprapubically exerts gentle upward pressure to keep the uterus in the abdomen while the right hand applies traction to the cord. Traction may be facilitated by winding the cord once around the fingers and the direction of its application follows the direction of the birth canal. Thus, with the patient lying on her back and the placenta still in utero, traction is applied in a downward and backward direction, and as the placenta descends into the vagina, the direction of pull curves upwards (Figure 30).

It is easy to appreciate that delivery of the placenta is being achieved normally and without the use of force, and if continuous progress is not being made either the direction of the pull is incorrect or the placenta has not separated adequately for delivery. As the membranes are being delivered they occasionally form a 'rope' which must be eased out of the birth canal in an upward direction. The last pieces of membrane should 'slither' or glide out of the vagina smoothly if delivered in their entirety.

The other normal method of placental delivery is that achieved by maternal effort. In this it is essential to wait for the placenta to descend into the vagina and with the next uterine contraction the patient flexes her hips and knees and 'bears down'. It is helpful to give the mother a resistance against which to push and rotate the hand which has been resting on the uterine fundus so that the palm exerts gentle pressure backwards over the area of the umbilicus. (The hand palpating the fundus not only enables the midwife to appreciate placental descent when it occurs, but also ensures that the uterus does not fill with blood).

At the earliest opportunity after delivery the placenta and membranes must be examined with care to ensure that they are complete. The fetal surface and membranes are inspected by first holding the placenta up by the cord. Blood vessels running across the fetal surface should disappear before reaching the placental edge and if torn vessels are found in the membranes, an accessory placenta or *succenturiate lobe* has been retained *in utero* and requires removal. A round hole in

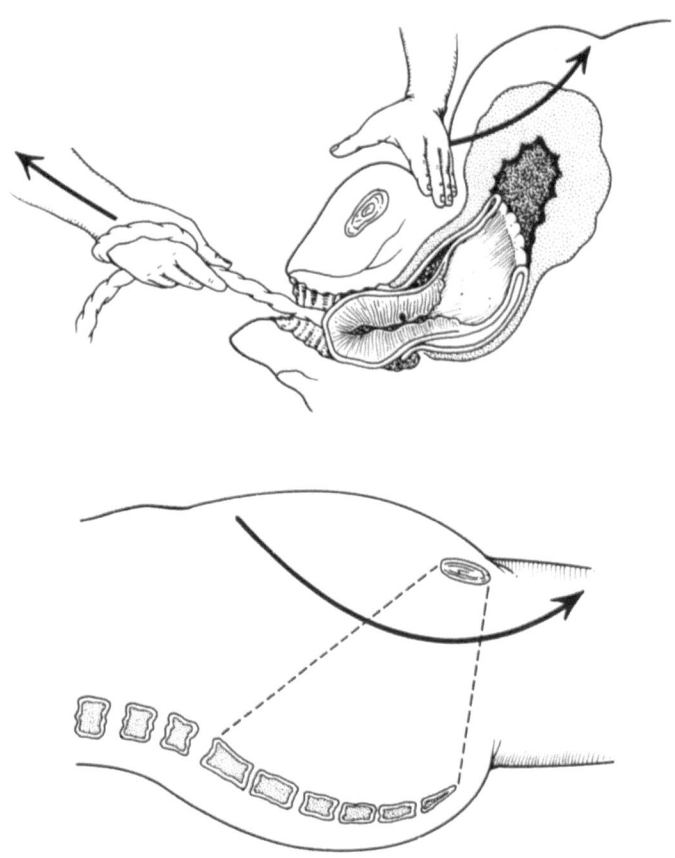

Figure 30   Cord traction in the third stage of labour

the membranes with a smooth edge usually indicates that they are complete. The maternal surface of the placenta is inspected by cupping it in both hands, but cotyledons should not be forced together when a roughened surface is being examined. Blood clot is removed by swabbing with gauze or with running water.

THE TREATMENT OF POSTPARTUM HAEMORRHAGE AND RETAINED PLACENTA

The essentials of the treatment of postpartum haemorrhage and retained placenta include:

(1)   Improving the patient's general condition.
(2)   Emptying the uterus.
(3)   Ensuring maintenance of normal uterine tone.

Treatment of the patient's general condition
This will include the replacement of blood loss by transfusion of whole blood or plasma expander such as dextran 70. The tendency to underestimate haemorrhage has been mentioned above and severe haemorrhagic (oligaemic) shock is best treated in intensive care conditions with monitoring of vital signs, central venous pressure and fluid charting. All patients who have sustained a heavy postpartum loss need reassurance and this should be given. Morphine is of value in most cases. The patient should be kept warm, but the use of hot water bottles in bed with her is to be avoided; they may be used to warm the bed but can burn a shocked patient whose peripheral circulation may be at a standstill.

Emptying the uterus
The placenta and membranes are delivered by:

(1)   Cord traction (sometimes referred to as the Brandt–Andrew method).
(2)   Expulsion by maternal effort.
       (1) and (2) are the normal methods described above.
(3)   Expulsion using the uterus as a 'piston'. During a contraction the fundus of the uterus is given a short sharp push with the ulnar border of the hand in a downward and backward direction. This will succeed only if the placenta has already descended, and the manoeuvre should not be necessary.
(4)   Expression of the uterus in an attempt to 'squeeze' out the retained placenta is obsolete and not without risk of increasing haemorrhage and shock. (I have not used Crede's expression for 30 years.)
(5)   *Manual removal.* Ideally this should be performed in a theatre with full aseptic and antiseptic facilities and with the patient under general anaesthesia. In emergency situations without these facilities it may be possible to explore a uterus with a patient sedated (by intravenous diazepam, for example) or even with no premedication. Practitioners have performed manual removal of the placenta after scrubbing their arms and covering them liberally with antiseptics. But of course the maternal risks are increased considerably where conditions are not ideal.

While the placenta remains in utero there is an ever-present risk of haemorrhage and it should be delivered within 60 minutes of the birth of the baby. Thus a midwife should summon medical aid if the third stage of labour has not been completed within 30 minutes, or earlier if there is any untoward bleeding.

In the majority of cases manual removal of the placenta is accomplished with ease, but occasionally difficulties are met, hence the need for general anaesthesia and operating theatre facilities. The patient's bladder is emptied, by catheter if necessary, and fresh sterile towels applied after cleansing the entire area. The patient is placed in the lithotomy position and access into the uterine cavity is obtained by following the cord through the cervix. When the edge of the placenta and its plane of separation have been identified, the obstetrician completes the separation by using a sawing motion of the whole right hand, fingers and thumb together and palmar surface facing the uterine cavity. Throughout the procedure the left hand placed on the patient's abdomen pushes the uterine fundus downward onto the internal hand. After placental separation is achieved, the uterus is massaged to 'rub-up' a contraction. The hand holding the placenta is removed as the uterus contracts. It is permissible to re-enter the uterine cavity once again to ensure that it is empty, but each reintroduction of the hand increases the risk of infection.

As the placenta is being extracted, an injection of an oxytocic agent is given. If a contraction ring is found, additional anaesthesia may be administered until the muscular spasm passes off. It is believed by some that inhalation of amyl nitrite (ampoules containing 3 to 5 minims of the volatile liquid are available) may relax a contraction ring, but this medication is usually ineffective.

Ensuring maintenance of normal uterine muscle tone
The injudicious use of oxytocic drugs and/or manipulation of the uterus (or 'fiddling'!) during the management of the third stage of labour are to be avoided and are listed among the more important causes of abnormal muscular irritability and contraction ring dystocia. Blood loss, however, must be kept to a minimum and when vaginal bleeding is associated with a relaxed, hypotonic uterus, a contraction may be stimulated by massage. If the placenta is still in the uterine cavity stimulation must be very gentle and is best performed by applying a gentle rotatory movement of the finger tips of the hand resting on the fundus. Stimulation of the myometrium after the placenta and membranes have been expelled may be more vigorous, but it is most important to ensure that the uterus remains high in the abdomen by exerting upward pressure with one hand placed suprapubically. If this is not observed and the hand massaging the fundus crowds the uterus into the pelvis, the organ will become engorged due to kinking

of the uterine blood vessels. Severe bleeding may occur through engorgement and this will cease as the uterus is raised out of the pelvis.

From the 1950s onward there was a remarkable drop in the number of maternal deaths in the United Kingdom from postpartum haemorrhage with retained placenta, and an important factor was the more frequent use of oxytocic drugs in labour. Thus, ergometrine 0.5 mg intramuscularly or 0.25 to 0.5 mg intravenously, possibly combined with oxytocin (5 units with 0.5 mg ergometrine in 1 ml ampoules – Syntometrine) are freely given. An injection may be given routinely in the second stage of labour after the anterior shoulder has been born (except where there is a possibility of multiple pregnancy) or after the third stage has been completed. An oxytocic injection should also be given if bleeding occurs during the third stage due to uterine hypotonicity, especially if a patient is being delivered in her own home. The hospital obstetrician can cope with a contraction ring which will rarely result, and the more important feature is the conservation of blood. Hospital emergency obstetric units ('flying squads') may be summoned by a nurse if required.

Massage of the uterus with one hand in the vaginal fornix and the other hand outside (*bimanual compression*) may sometimes be indicated to control haemorrhage associated with the hypotonic uterus. Intrauterine packs are usually better avoided but may be necessary. Finally (and hopefully very rarely indeed), hysterectomy or ligation of the internal iliac arteries may be considered where bleeding is otherwise uncontrollable.

Secondary postpartum haemorrhage may be due to causes mentioned above, but is often associated with retained products of conception and infection. Evacuation of the uterus under antibiotic cover may be required. Living chorionic tissue in the uterus will produce chorionic gonadotrophin (HCG) and if this is present a few weeks postpartum (in other words a pregnancy test is positive) the remote possibility of chorioncarcinoma should be considered.

OTHER CAUSES OF POSTPARTUM SHOCK
Postpartum haematomata
Bleeding into the subcutaneous and submucous tissues of the vulva and vagina may occasionally be extensive and cause considerable pain, without an obvious excessive vaginal loss. A tense haematoma may be visible or be felt bulging into the vagina on examination with one finger. Expectant treatment may suffice but often evacuation of the haematoma and ligation of the bleeding points under general anaesthesia is required. Antibiotic cover is advisable.

Rupture of the uterus
This is dealt with in Chapter 19 on obstructed labour.

Acute inversion of the uterus
The uterus may be turned inside out, especially when hypotonic and fundal pressure and cord traction have been unwisely used. This is a rare complication and is reputed to be associated with shock, although this was not marked in the few cases I have seen. The uterus may be replaced by applying digital pressure or hydrostatically with warm sterile water poured into the vagina. Uterine packing after replacement may help.

Bacteraemic or endotoxic shock
This is associated with infection by Gram-negative bacteria, such as *Escherichia coli* (see also page 205).

Pulmonary embolism
This is dealt with in Chapter 24.

8

The mechanisms of labour

Mechanisms of labour describe, but do not necessarily explain, the movements made by the fetus during its passage through the birth canal in labour. Before a detailed consideration of individual mechanisms is made, certain fundamental facts may be noted:

(1)   The normal attitude of the fetus *in utero* is one of full flexion — that is the head is flexed on the trunk, and the upper and lower limbs are fully flexed.

(2)   The fetal spine is not twisted before the onset of labour.

(3)   A rotatory movement of the fetus within the birth canal is described as *internal rotation*, while *external rotation* takes place outside the mother's pelvis. Thus, in the second stage of labour when the baby's shoulders rotate inside the pelvis, the head, if lying completely free outside, will be carried round to the same extent. This internal rotation of the shoulders is manifest as external rotation of the head.

In about 90% of vertex presentations the fetal head enters the pelvis with its occiput lying opposite the iliopectineal eminence or more laterally. During labour, however, the occiput usually rotates to the front so that it emerges from the maternal pelvis immediately below the symphysis pubis. Internal rotation of the occiput occurs because in the normal delivery where the head is fully flexed the occiput is the most dependent part of the fetus and reaches the pelvic floor first. The muscles of the latter form a gutter or sling, the upper surface of which points upwards, forwards and towards the midline (page 22). Thus as descent of the head occurs during labour the occiput is directed to the front.

Understanding the mechanisms of labour means that the midwife knows what is taking place during delivery and anticipates the next step in the birth process. This understanding promotes better management. The mechanisms are described below with the aid of diagrams of the maternal pelvic inlet (Figures 31, 32 and 33). Although certain diameters may require memorizing, little else does, and features may be readily appreciated if one imagines the fetus to be passing or diving through the pelvis as depicted. Before labour commences, the diameter occupied by the shoulders must be diametrically opposed to that occupied by the occiput and sinciput. Furthermore, shoulders must be in the same plane as the hips. In normal labour, as fetal descent occurs, the head enters the maternal pelvis and the occiput rotates to the front. The shoulders follow and the anterior one rotates to the front in turn. In a breech delivery, the buttocks, or hips, enter the pelvis and the anterior one rotates to the front, then the shoulders do likewise, and lastly the head enters the pelvis and the occiput rotates to the front as described below.

In the figures illustrating mechanisms, rotatory movements are indicated by arrows, those drawn inside the pelvis represent internal rotation, and those outside the pelvis represent external rotation.

The vertex presentation in the left occipito-anterior (LOA) position
The left occipito-anterior is the most common position adopted by the fetus at the onset of labour. The use of the term LOA to describe the position implies that the fetal lie must be longitudinal, the presentation cephalic and the head flexed so that the vertex presents, and that the denominator, the occiput, is entering the pelvis opposite the left iliopectineal eminence (Figure 31). For diagrammatic purposes the sinciput is shown to be more pointed than the occiput and the shoulders are represented by small circles.

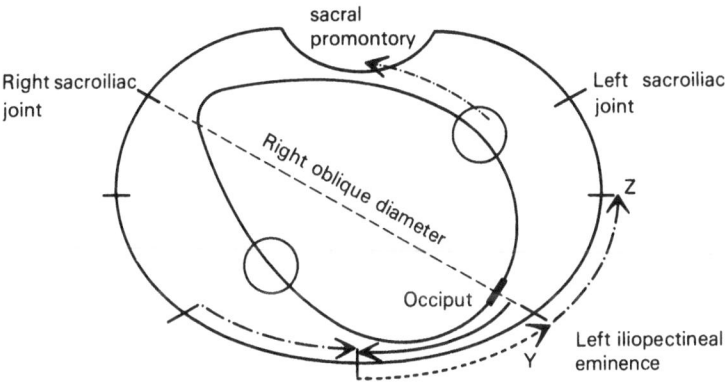

Figure 31   Mechanism of labour, left occipito-anterior (LAO) position

The following steps take place in the delivery of the fetus in the left occipito-anterior position (see Figure 31). Fetal descent is continuous.

(1)   *Engagement.* The suboccipito-bregmatic diameter (9.5 cm) engages in the right oblique diameter of the pelvic inlet.

(2)   *Internal rotation of the occiput,* as the occiput reaches the pelvic floor and rotates to the front through one-eighth of a circle. This means that the baby's neck has twisted (internal rotation is shown thus ⤺).

(3)   As further descent occurs, the occipital protuberance emerges under the symphysis pubis (as the head is 'crowned'), and the head is born by *extension* as sinciput, face and chin appear over the perineum.

(4)   *Restitution* occurs (one-eighth of a circle). When the head is free, the neck untwists and the occiput returns to position Y (restitution is shown thus ....⤴).

(5)   At this stage the shoulders enter the pelvis in the left oblique diameter, and the anterior rotates to the front (one-eighth of a circle) and appears in the subpubic arch, followed by the posterior shoulder born posteriorly over the perineum. This movement of *internal rotation* of the shoulders is transmitted to the head which rotates externally so that the occiput arrives at point Z, or facing the mother's left thigh (internal rotation of shoulders and external rotation of occiput are shown thus ._.⤴).

(6)   The birth of the posterior shoulder and the trunk of the baby is accompanied by *lateral flexion of the spine* as the process is completed and the baby is born following the curve of the birth canal.

OCCIPITO-POSTERIOR POSITIONS

In approximately 10% of vertex presentations the occiput is posteriorly placed and more often when this is so it enters the pelvis in the region of the right sacroiliac joint. The occipito-posterior position occurs because either the head is incompletely flexed, or the shape of the pelvic inlet is such that the head best fits with the wider occipital area posteriorly (see anthropoid pelvis, Figure 47, page 168). It should be stressed, however, that the head is in an attitude of flexion, albeit incomplete, so that the presentation is that of a vertex. Clinical aspects are discussed below but the mechanism may follow that described for the occipito-anterior position with one added feature, that of engagement taking place in two stages. The incompletely flexed head at the onset of labour enters the pelvis with longer diameters engaging, but usually full flexion occurs as labour progresses. If this takes place (step (2) in the mechanism below) spontaneous delivery is likely.

The fetus in the right occipito-posterior (ROP) position
The lie is longitudinal, presentation cephalic in attitude of incomplete flexion, and the occiput enters the pelvis opposite the right sacroiliac joint (Figure 32).

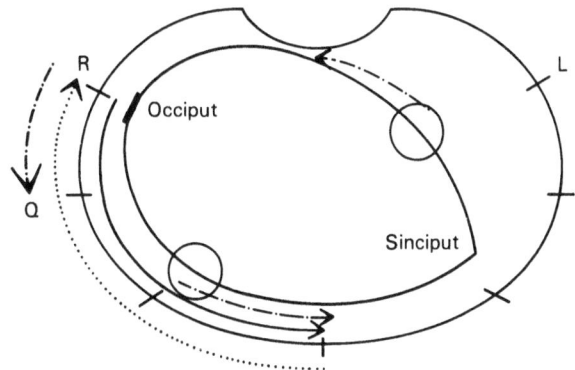

Figure 32 Mechanism of labour, right occipito-posterior (ROP) position

The following steps take place:

(1) *Engagement.* The head enters the pelvis incompletely flexed, with either suboccipito-frontal (10 cm) or occipito-frontal (11 cm) diameter engaging in the right oblique diameter of the pelvis.
(2) As descent of the head progresses in labour, usually full flexion occurs, so that the diameter of engagement becomes suboccipito-bregmatic (9.5 cm). The mechanism may then follow that described on page 88 – (3), (4), (5), and (6).
(3) *Internal rotation of the occiput* to the front is associated with a twist of the neck through three-eighths of a circle (arrow ⟍→).
(4) As further descent of the head takes place, the occiput appears below the symphysis pubis and crowning is followed by the birth of the head by extension.
(5) *Restitution* occurs (three-eighths of a circle) as the massive twist on the baby's neck unwinds and the occiput returns to position R (⟵······).
(6) Shoulders enter pelvis in left oblique diameter and rotate internally (one-eighth circle). The anterior shoulder rotates to the front and appears in subpubic angle followed by the birth of the posterior shoulder over the perineum. *Internal rotation of the shoulders* causes external rotation of the occiput to point Q (⟍).
(7) Posterior shoulder and rest of baby are born accompanied by *lateral flexion of the spine.*

COMMON MODIFICATION OF MECHANISM (ROP POSITION)
The above mechanism of labour is associated with considerable rotation of the fetal neck, and so it is often modified in the following manner. As internal rotation of the occiput through three-eighths of a circle takes place, the shoulders and trunk of the fetus rotate at the same time through two-eighths of a circle thereby relieving the twist of the baby's neck. The shoulders thus eventually occupy the right oblique diameter of the pelvis instead of the left. Restitution will now be through only one-eighth of a circle and with external rotation of the occiput as shown (Figure 33) it arrives at the same lateral point Q. Other features of the mechanism remain unchanged.

The description of rotatory movements through eighths of a circle may appear to be more appropriate to a textbook on mathematics rather than obstetrics. It is, however, apt and reasonable to suppose that as the occiput rotates through three-eighths of a circle, the trunk and shoulders are carried round to a lesser extent due to the resistance met.

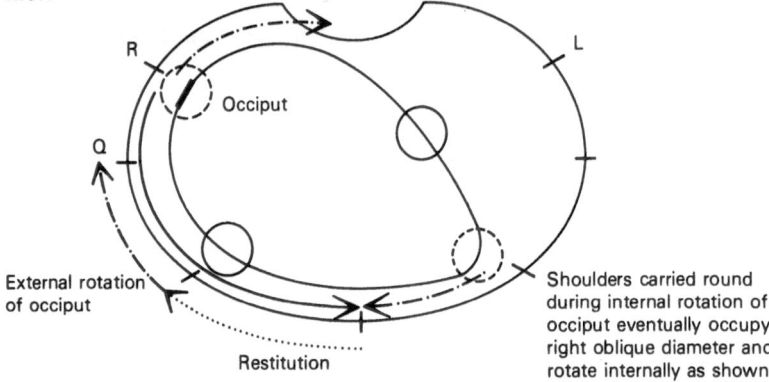

Figure 33   Common modification of mechanism, right occipito-posterior (ROP) position

Clinical features of occipito-posterior position
The following clinical features found prenatally suggest that the fetus is in an occipito-posterior position.

(1)   The contour of the abdomen. A scaphoid depression may sometimes be felt above the head suprapubically because of the absence of the firm broad curved fetal back.
(2)   The fetal back is felt well out in the mother's flank.
(3)   Limbs are prominent on both sides of the uterus.
(4)   The fetal heart is generally most clearly audible over its back (in the maternal flank). However, occasionally it is best heard in

the midline (over the fetal chest) and especially when the head is very poorly flexed.

(5) Non-engagement of the head in the last weeks of pregnancy. This is associated with deficient flexion which may be appreciated on abdominal palpation by finding that the occiput and sinciput are at the same level. This sign is of more significance in primigravidae in whom a posterior position of the fetus should be suspected if the head is not engaged by the 38th week of pregnancy.

(6) *Vaginal examination.* The positive diagnosis of occipito-posterior position is made by vaginal examination which is usually performed early in the first stage of labour. When any such examination is made, the midwife notes;

(a) the state of the vagina;
(b) the station of the head and whether moulding or caput succadeneum is present;
(c) the condition and degree of dilatation of the cervix;
(d) whether the membranes are intact;
(e) whether the umbilical cord can be felt;
(f) the fetal position;
(g) the degree of flexion of the head.

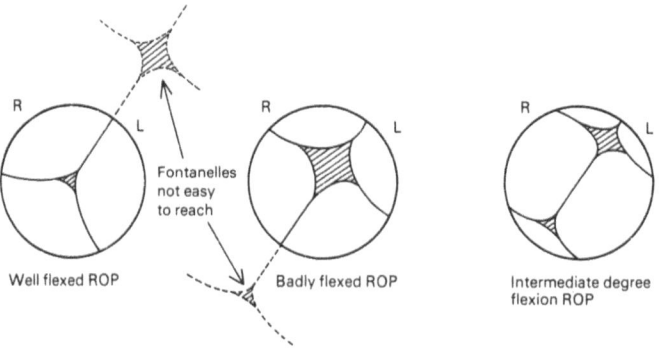

Figure 34 'Touch' pictures of vaginal examination findings in labour with patient in lithiotomy position

The circles in Figure 34 represent the area most easily explored vaginally with two fingers and with the patient placed in the lithotomy position. Identification of the posterior fontanelle shows that in each case the occiput is posterior and to the mother's right (that is, the ROP position). If the posterior fontanelle is felt most easily, the head is well flexed, and if the anterior fontanelle is most prominent, the head is badly flexed.

If forward rotation of the occiput fails to occur in labour the following may take place:

(1)   The occiput may rotate backwards to the hollow of the maternal sacrum and a *persistent occipito-posterior* position (POP) result. Spontaneous face-to-pubis delivery may occur in which either

(a)   the badly flexed head is forced down so that the forehead is born below the symphysis followed by flexion as the head pivots by the root of the nose around the pubic arch, or

(b)   marked flexion occurs, the occiput escapes over the perineum and the head is born by extension as face and brow appear behind the pubis.

An experienced observer may deduce that a face-to-pubis delivery is taking place, as early in the second stage there is marked projection on the perineum causing the anus to gape and perineal body to stretch long before anticipated crowning of the head. A liberal episiotomy (see page 102) is usually indicated. The first stage of labour, too, is often prolonged and the patient has a more severe low backache than she might be expected to have if the fetus were in an occipito-anterior position.

(2)   *Deep transverse arrest* may occur. In this, the deflexed head is forced downwards and the occiput and sinciput arrive at the pelvic floor together. Therefore, neither can rotate anteriorly and a 'stalemate' condition results. The head impacts in the pelvis at the level of the ischial spines and vaginal examination reveals the sagittal suture lying transversely. The patient usually requires assistance.

(3)   A badly flexed head in the occipito-posterior position may extend into a brow or face. The latter may be born spontaneously.

PROGNOSIS

Over 80% of labours that commence with the fetus in the occipito-posterior position terminate by spontaneous vaginal delivery; 70% or more rotate naturally to an anterior position and about another 10% deliver face-to-pubis. Spontaneous deliveries increase with the correct use of intravenous oxytocic infusions in labour. Assistance when required may take the form of;

(1)   Rotation of the head to an anterior position and extraction with Kielland's forceps.
(2)   Manual rotation and forceps extraction.
(3)   Forceps extraction as face-to-pubis.
(4)   Ventouse (or vacuum) extraction.
(5)   Caesarean section.

9

The management of labour

The management of labour commences at a patient's first prenatal consultation and the importance of confidence, knowledge and preparation for childbirth has been discussed above (page 46). When admitted in early labour, a patient's records are obtained and studied and she is asked to give her history of the onset of labour. Records are made of the time contractions commenced, their frequency and strength on admission, and whether there has been a 'show' or loss of blood or liquor. Pulse rate, temperature and blood pressure are recorded, the patient empties her bladder and the specimen of urine is examined. The abdomen is palpated, the fetal heart checked and the patient is told if all is well. It is usual to offer the patient a shower and empty the lower bowel with suppositories or an enema. Routine practices may differ but for some years in my units shaving has not been performed although pudendal hair if abundant may be trimmed with scissors. Vaginal examination is usual but not invariable (see page 50).

It is important also for the midwife to observe the general appearance and demeanour of the patient, and if prenatal preparation has achieved its aim one hopes to find the expectant mother looking forward to having her baby. However, there is often an element of anxiety concerning labour itself, the drugs or methods that may be used to alleviate discomfort and the possible effects they may have on the patient herself and the baby. Will the baby survive and be normal, and may her husband remain with her, are some of the questions that concern the patient. Procedures to be performed and the principles of management are discussed and it is often desirable and useful for nurse and patient to chat during preparatory procedures.

The first stage

The first stage of labour may be divided into a *latent phase*, which lasts from the onset of regular contractions, until the *active phase*

commences when the cervix dilates from 3 cm. Since the exact timing
of the start of labour is often difficult to pinpoint, observations made
will not necessarily follow a precisely set routine. However, the important features to consider in the management of the first stage of labour
are:

(1)   The maternal physical condition.
(2)   The maternal psychological condition.
(3)   That progress is continuous and satisfactory and will end in
safe vaginal delivery.
(4)   That the fetal condition remains satisfactory.

MATERNAL PHYSICAL CONDITION
Comfort and nourishment are two important considerations here. The
patient's temperature and blood pressure are recorded every 2 to 4
hours and pulse rate at least ½-hourly during the active phase of
labour. Overdistension of the bladder is a cause of delay in the first
stage of labour and should be avoided by encouraging the patient to
void urine at least 4 hourly. Each specimen passed must be tested for
protein and acetone. If ketonuria is present, and especially if accompanied by evidence of dehydration (such as dry tongue, or hot and dry
vagina), an intravenous infusion of 500 ml or more of 10% glucose is
administered.

If there is no obvious risk of prolapsed cord and the membranes are
intact, the patient may be up and about if she so desires during the
latent phase. When labour is proceeding actively she will prefer to be
in bed but should lie well propped up with pillows, or on her side. She
must not adopt the supine attitude, a posture which in late pregnancy
may cause hypotension and faintness because pressure of the uterus
on the inferior vena cava obstructs the venous return to the heart
(*supine hypotensive syndrome*). Furthermore, such hypotension will
reduce the placental blood supply, and labour itself is an anoxic
process for the fetus as the uterus contracts and retracts on the
placental site.

Oral feeding is better avoided in active labour, and the patient's
mouth may be kept comfortable by moistening her lips with water or
giving her ice to suck. Although additional energy requirements for
labour are met basically by using glucose, its administration orally is
contraindicated during active labour when the gastric emptying time is
markedly prolonged. If liquid gastric contents are regurgitated and
inhaled, as can occur during or following anaesthesia, the patient
might develop *Mendelson's syndrome*. In this condition, after a latent
period of 1 to 3 hours, gross pulmonary oedema occurs, when as a
reaction to the acid gastric juices inhaled the bronchiolar mucosa and

pulmonary capillaries exude large amounts of fluid. For this reason it is a good routine, especially where the first stage of labour is prolonged, to give the patient a simple alkaline mixture such as 15 ml magnesium trisilicate, every 2 or 3 hours to neutralize gastric acidity.

Sedation and the relief of pain, if and when required, should be adequate and this subject is dealt with separately (page 98).

MATERNAL PSYCHOLOGICAL CONDITION

The anxieties of an expectant mother, and the importance of confidence in herself and in her midwifery team have been stressed many times above. Individuals differ in their reactions physically and psychologically and the midwife must always bear this in mind. All who help to look after obstetric patients will meet the very occasional women and/or her husband who may be 'demanding' or 'difficult' but even this very small minority will usually respond to a professional and understanding approach.

PROGRESS IN THE FIRST STAGE

Provided maternal and fetal conditions remain satisfactory, normal progress in the first stage of labour entails normal uterine activity associated with progressive dilatation of the cervix and descent of the head. The latter is determined by both abdominal palpation and vaginal examination in which the station or depth of the head in the pelvis may be related to the ischial spines. An excessive degree of moulding or caput formation, or failure of the vertex to flex fully,.should alert the midwife to possible difficulties in labour (dystocia).

THE FETAL CONDITION

The fetal heart rate if not monitored continuously must be recorded at least ½-hourly during active labour, and often every 15 minutes or more frequently. If there is any concern, or if liquor is stained with meconium, the fetal heart rate should be counted during and after every contraction. The normal rate varies between 120 and 160 beats per minute (bpm), and a rate of below 100 or above 180 is a positive indication of fetal distress. The heart may slow during a contraction (type 1 deceleration in monitoring) but should regain normal rate and rhythm within a short time. Slowing of the heart rate occurring after the contraction has passed (type 2 deceleration in monitoring) or the passage of meconium-stained liquor indicates the need for increased observation of the fetal heart. Convulsive fetal movements, or faintness of the heart sound, although not to be disregarded, are less important in detecting fetal distress than an alteration in rate or rhythm of the heart beat. A variation of more than 20 bpm from the normal rate merits the most careful and continuous observation while preparations for urgent delivery are made. Oxygen administration to the mother, who must be lying on her side, is often of value.

The partogram: active management and monitoring in labour
The partogram used in some maternity units is a composite graphical record made to show progress in labour. The form it takes differs but most partographical records show:

(1)   The maternal condition (pulse rate, blood pressure, urine tests and temperature).
(2)   The fetal condition (heart rate, state of liquor, degree of moulding and caput).
(3)   The uterine contractions (frequency and duration).
(4)   Any treatment or intravenous fluids given.
(5)   The descent of the fetal head.
(6)   The state of the cervix.

Regular vaginal examinations – at least every 4 hours – are performed during the active phase of labour and the graph should show at a glance whether the cervix is dilating normally. It is considered that the cervix should dilate at the rate of at least 1 cm per hour in a primigravida and 1.5 cm per hour in the multipara.

In so-called active management of labour where maternal and fetal conditions remain satisfactory but progress in the first stage appears to be delayed, a most careful re-evaluation of every factor is necessary. If the latent phase exceeds 8 hours, or cervical dilatation or descent of the fetal head is not progressing as described in the last paragraph, the membranes may be ruptured artificially and an oxytocic infusion commenced (see induction of labour, Chapter 21). The intact bag of forewaters provides an effective barrier against infection, but very tough membranes will cause delay. Every experienced midwife has seen cases in which artificial rupture of the forewaters has accelerated the first stage and also given the patient relief from some pain.

The partogram may provide a useful pictorial record of progress in labour and if accurately kept will alert the obstetrician to deviations from normality. Labour, however, does not progress with mathematical precision, and the estimation, for example, of the exact number of fifths of the head above the pelvic inlet may vary with the observer (and also with the state of the bladder) and these factors, too, must be remembered. Active management is best practised where there are facilities for monitoring processes, including uterine contractions (tocography), the fetal heart rate, and fetal blood sampling.

UTERINE CONTRACTIONS

Means of monitoring uterine contractions may be either:

(1) *External*, by strapping a transducer to the abdominal wall. This is a diaphragm with a small central movable plunger and provides a means of recording the movements of the uterine wall and hence the uterine contractions on a paper trace.

(2) *Internal*, with recording devices passed into the uterus transvaginally or via the abdominal wall. These measure changes of pressure within the uterus converting them to a line on a paper recorder and again producing a record of uterine contractions.

THE FETAL HEART RATE

This may be monitored either:

(1) *Externally*, by ultrasonic techniques. The transducer is strapped to the abdominal wall.

(2) *Internally*. A direct electrocardiographic recording can be made after the membranes have ruptured, and monitoring maintained if necessary until the child is delivered. A spiral or clip electrode is attached to the fetal scalp and the fetal ECG recorded on a moving strip of graph paper.

The external monitors above mentioned are easy to apply but they are less reliable as they may move when the mother moves. The internal devices are more reliable if accurately placed, but they involve certain risks such as haemorrhage or infection, and they may be less acceptable to the patient. Acceptability or otherwise of all equipment must be considered.

FETAL BLOOD SAMPLING

A sample of blood may be obtained from the fetal scalp with a tiny guarded scalpel. This is examined for pH value (acidity) and oxygen content. The test is performed selectively when there are other indications of possible fetal distress. Fetal acidosis is sought as a confirmation of distress and may indicate the need for urgent delivery. It may be associated with maternal acidosis or hypoxia. Recently, continuous recordings of tissue pH in the fetal scalp have been made; these do not require repeated blood sampling.

Oxytocin intravenous drips are discussed in Chapter 21 on induction of labour. The drip rate can be electronically controlled, and when attached to an automatic infusion system may alter according to the strength and frequency of the uterine contractions.

Relief of pain in labour
DRUGS
Drugs for the relief of pain in labour are not given routinely and the patient's own desires are of importance. If preparation methods for childbirth have been satisfactorily used, the expectant mother often requires less sedation and analgesia. Some women may prefer to have no drug therapy whatsoever to ensure they do not 'lose self-control'. Drugs used for sedation and the relief of pain include the following.

Chloral hydrate and dichloral-phenazone (Welldorm 650 mg tablets × 2)
These sedatives and hypnotics are not used as often as they were decades ago. Chloral hydrate mixtures had a ghastly taste and over 30 years ago midwives often administered the drug rectally! The drugs may be secreted in breast milk and may cause minimal sedation in the neonate.

Barbiturates
Barbiturates are better avoided. Their safety in pregnancy has not been established, and individual reaction to barbiturates is very variable.

Morphine
Morphine 10 to 15 mg by injection causes respiratory depression in the fetus and should not be given if delivery is anticipated within 4 hours. An allied preparation, papaveretum (Omnopon) 20 mg is a mixture of opium alkaloids and less likely to cause nausea and vomiting.

Pethidine and levallorphan
Pethidine 100, 150 or even 200 mg by injection is commonly used and may be repeated after 3 to 4 hours if necessary. It also depresses the fetal respiratory centre and should be avoided if delivery within 1 hour is expected. Ampoules containing 50 mg pethidine with 0.625 mg of levallorphan tartrate (Lorfan) are available and may be used in doses of 1 or 2 ml.

Levallorphan is a narcotic antagonist and reduces the respiratory depressant effect of the injection. It may be administered directly to the infant with drug-induced respiratory depression, 0.25 mg intravenously, as may naloxone (Narcan) 0.01 mg/kg (body weight) intravenously initially, or a single dose of 200 μg intramuscularly only.

Phenothiazine derivatives
The use of these drugs is better avoided during lactation and pregnancy, especially in the earlier months. Promazine (Sparine) 50 mg

intramuscularly may be combined with 50 mg pethidine for use in labour and will combine sedative and antiemetic effects. Promethazine (Phenergan) 25 to 50 mg intramuscularly is a long-acting antihistamine which has a similar action, and chlorpromazine (Largactil) 25 to 50 mg intramuscularly is used occasionally when a patient is in active labour.

Diazepam (Valium)
Diazepam has anxiolytic and anticonvulsant properties (see Chapter 15 on eclampsia). Ampoules for intravenous use contain 10 mg in 2 ml, and slow injection (0.5 ml in 30 seconds) may sedate adequately for minor surgical procedures. Neonatal hypotonia is reported and the fetal level of the drug exceeds maternal level. Although this may not be harmful a few obstetricians prefer not to use it.

Pentazocine (Fortral)
This is an analgesic recommended by some as an alternative to pethidine. It is said to cause psychotic reactions, but I have no personal experience of its use.

Personal preference in recent years has been for pethidine, the phenothiazine derivatives and diazepam.

SELF-ADMINISTERED INHALATION ANALGESICS
The machines which enable a patient in labour to inhale analgesic vapours via a face mask should have been demonstrated to her in parentcraft classes, and when they are to be used in labour the midwife initially supervises the administration. The gases are inhaled as the contraction builds up and the mask is discarded between contractions. As the onset of analgesia is delayed for several seconds the gases should be taken as an anticipatory measure. Machines used include Entonox and Emotril apparatuses.

Entonox apparatus
This administers equal quantities of nitrous oxide and oxygen. The 50% of oxygen in the mixture increases the oxygen supply to the fetus, so this is one of the best inhalation analgesics.

Emotril apparatus
The Emotril provides 0.5% of trichloroethylene (Trilene) vapour in air (and the Tecota 0.35%). Trichloroethylene is eliminated from the body more slowly than nitrous oxide and the apparatus should not be used for more than 4 hours. Excessive use may cause the patient to become confused temporarily. Full inhalation analgesia is better em-

ployed late in the first stage and during the second stage of labour. Methoxyflurane (Penthrane) has replaced trichloroethylene in some units.

EPIDURAL ANALGESIA

A local anaesthetic, bupivacaine (Marcain) 0.5%, is introduced into the epidural space when labour is established. A Tuohy needle is used and it is important to ensure that the subarachnoid space has not been entered (no cerebrospinal fluid should escape). Initially a small test dose of bupivacaine is injected, and if no untoward reaction occurs, 8 ml of the agent is given. A plastic tube threaded through the needle is left *in situ* for top-up purposes.

If successful, epidural analgesia will give complete relief from pain and the patient remains fully conscious. Hypotension may occur and the patient must be nursed on her side and her blood pressure checked regularly. Collapse occurs if the anaesthetic passes into the subarachnoid space, and the setting up of an intravenous infusion before administering an epidural block is a wise precaution. Other side-effects of epidural anaesthesia include nausea and headache. Assisted vaginal delivery, usually forceps extraction, is more common in these cases but analgesia is achieved with no associated depression of the infant's respiratory centre. This analgesia is of special value in pre-eclampsia and heart disease and in cases of incoordinate uterine action (pages 144 and 180).

Epidural analgesia should be administered by specialist anaesthetists or obstetricians skilled in this technique with trained nursing staff at hand to keep the patient under constant observation.

PUDENDAL NERVE BLOCK

This is used largely for low forceps delivery and also as a preliminary to breech delivery if epidural analgesia has not been given. The pudendal nerve supplies areas of the lower vagina, perineum, labia majora. and the superficial perineal muscles. These zones may be made insensitive by injecting up to 10 ml of 0.5% lignocaine around the nerve on each side as it crosses the ischial spine. The latter is identified by palpation on vaginal examination and the local anaesthetic is injected behind and below this point. An additional 10 ml is used to infiltrate the subcutaneous tissues of the perineum and the lower half of the labia. Approach to the area of the spine may be from the perineal region or transvaginally with a special needle and guard to control the depth of injection. Aspiration prior to injection will ensure that a blood vessel has not been entered.

PARACERVICAL BLOCK

This is sometimes used late in the first stage of labour. The recommended dose is 10 ml of 0.25% bupivacaine injected with a guarded needle via the lateral fornices into the tissues at the sides of the cervix where the nerve plexuses are situated. I have personally not used this method but it is said to be helpful in the active phase of the first stage when the cervix is at least 5 cm dilated.

The second stage

The midwife will often be aware of the fact that the patient's cervix is fully dilated and that she is ready to deliver the baby without performing an examination. Uterine contractions when this stage is reached are generally strong and occurring at less than 5 minute intervals, and in an ideal labour the membranes rupture spontaneously. The timing of the latter does, however, vary considerably and it should be noted that spontaneous rupture of the forewaters early in the first stage, especially with a malpresentation (see Chapter 10), may be a bad prognostic sign. As the fetal head reaches the pelvic floor the patient's reaction to a contraction changes and bearing down becomes involuntary. Spasm of the glottis and contraction of the abdominal musculature is usually accompanied by facial congestion and grunting. Delivery should take place with the patient in the position she finds most comfortable, initially perhaps on her left side and as delivery approaches on her back. Recently the ancient method of squatting for delivery has been revived, a posture which I feel has its advantages. Inhalation analgesia may be used as required. The fetal heart is noted after each contraction and maternal pulse rate is checked at least every 15 minutes.

The mother who is now 'labouring' in every sense of the word, should know precisely what to expect and what is expected of her. If there is any doubt concerning the state of the cervix a vaginal examination must be performed to ensure that there is full dilatation, as premature bearing down will cause oedema of the cervix and may lead to difficulties. When the patient bears down with hips and knees flexed, the perineum bulges and soon an area of the fetal scalp becomes visible. The perineal body thins out and the anus gapes. Maternal efforts are more effective if the push is sustained and this is aided by the patient breathing in deeply before bearing down. She should be encouraged to relax between contractions, and she is kept informed of progress by the midwife who must remain with the patient constantly. The expectant father can be a member of the patient–midwife team by passing on to his wife the midwife's instructions and encouragement.

The woman must not bear down during a contraction when the head is about to crown and be born by extension, as delivery would be too rapid and possibly rupture the perineum. The irresistible urge to push down can be overcome by the patient panting rapidly and audibly in and out through her mouth. When the contraction has passed, a gentle effort by the mother should effect controlled delivery of the head. When the baby's head has been delivered the air passages are cleared, usually by sucking out secretions from nose and mouth. A digital examination is made to check the umbilical cord is not wound around the baby's neck or otherwise obstructing the delivery of the shoulders. If cord is found and is loosely applied it may be slipped over the shoulders gently. Occasionally, if the cord is very tightly wound around the neck, it may be necessary to cut it between two haemostatic forceps.

When the anterior shoulder has been born, an intramuscular or intravenous injection of ergometrine (with or without oxytocin, see page 84) is of value in preventing haemorrhage and delay in the third stage of labour. The administration of this oxytocic drug is contraindicated if there is another fetus still in utero or there is a history of allergy to the drug. The posterior shoulder and trunk are eased out of the birth canal accompanied by lateral flexion of the spine as described in the mechanism.

In the second stage of labour the midwife's function is to encourage the mother and to ensure that she and her baby come to no harm. By controlling a natural delivery, damage to the perineum and its musculature, the vaginal mucosa and labia may be prevented. Episiotomy may be indicated (*as below*). The careful employment of aseptic and antiseptic techniques will guard against infection.

Episiotomy
A clean cut made with a scissors through the tissues of the perineum when indicated, and if performed at the correct time, can be of great value to mother and baby. Indeed, as far as the latter is concerned, the procedure may be a life-saving one. Indications for episiotomy are as follows.

FETAL INDICATIONS
    (1)   Preterm delivery. To prevent intracranial damage due to pressure of the pelvic floor on the immature skull.
    (2)   Multiple pregnancy. For similar reasons as (1).
    (3)   Breech delivery. For reasons as above and to facilitate delivery of the aftercoming head.

(4)   To hasten delivery in the second stage of labour if fetal distress becomes apparent for any reason.

(5)   To release the head of any fetus when held up on the perineum. Prolonged pressure increases the risks even at full term.

MATERNAL INDICATIONS

(1)   A rigid perineum or one with excessive scar tissue from old tears.

(2)   If the perineum appears to be in danger of splitting.

(3)   Previous pelvic floor repair operations.

METHOD

Episiotomies may be mediolateral (straight or 'J'-shaped) or midline. The latter has its advocates as the area is less vascular and a natural tear tends to occur in this direction which suggests that it is the area of maximal muscle resistance. However, most prefer to direct the cut away from the anus and rectum, and personal preference is for the straight mediolateral incision (Figure 35). Bilateral episiotomy is very rarely necessary.

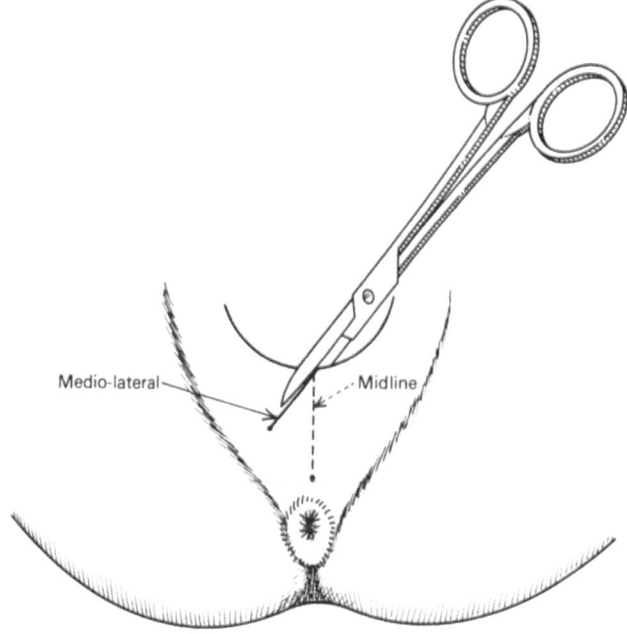

Figure 35   Episiotomy, mediolateral and midline

In an emergency the operation can be performed without anaes-thesia, especially if the patient is having inhalation analgesia. A few rapid deep inspirations of, say, gas and oxygen, and a solitary cut with a scissors at the height of a contraction will usually leave no painful impression. However, normally local anaesthetic (0.5 or 1% ligno-caine) should be used. The needle is inserted in the midline of the four-chette, or through torn skin if present, and passed subcutaneously to a point about 1 cm beyond the end of the intended cut. Initial aspiration should ensure that a blood vessel has not been entered, after which the lignocaine is injected as the needle is withdrawn to raise a subcutan-eous bleb. An additional amount of 1 to 2 ml of anaesthetic is injected at the mucocutaneous junction and for a short distance under the vag-inal mucosa.

The episiotomy scissors, blunt-pointed but sharp-bladed, are directed into position between two fingers inserted into the vagina. At the height of a contraction a solitary cut through vaginal mucosa, skin and perineal body should suffice. Occasionally a thin band of uncut muscle may warrant an immediate second cut, but one, and not more than two, incisions should suffice. When the procedure is properly timed immediate delivery of the head should follow.

Occasionally it is necessary to perform an early episiotomy when the pelvic floor appears to hold up progress in the second stage before the head is about to crown. If bleeding results from the procedure, gentle pressure with a sterile swab or cotton wool pledget applied between contractions should stop the loss. Pressure is removed during a con-traction. Rarely, a haemostatic forceps may be applied to stop loss from a small artery.

10

Breech presentations

Causes of malpresentations

In over 95% of pregnancies the fetus at term will present head first whether or not the expectant mother has had prenatal care. This is because the fetus in its normal attitude of full flexion fits best into the uterus in this way. This is particularly so because in the latter weeks of pregnancy the uterus undergoes painless contractions (Braxton—Hicks) which tend to make the longitudinal axis of the passenger align itself with that of the passage. The broad fetal back needs more room than the ventral surface and tends to occupy the anterior half of the uterus, as the maternal lumbar spine projects into the posterior portion of her abdomen. In the last weeks of pregnancy the head may engage in the pelvis.

Causes of malpresentations in general may be classified in various ways, and the following has been found most useful.

Fetal causes
(1)   Prematurity: maceration: multiple pregnancy.
(2)   Anencephaly; hydrocephaly.
(3)   Hydramnios.
(4)   Placenta praevia.

Maternal causes
(1)   Contracted pelvis.
(2)   Pelvic tumours (such as fibroids).
(3)   Grand multiparity associated with a 'pendulous belly'.
(4)   Developmental abnormalities of the uterus.

This list should be memorized and considered whenever a malpresentation is found. Usually, however, no obvious cause is immediately apparent and this is discussed further under individual malpresentations.

Breech presentation

Abdominal palpation at the 30th week of pregnancy to ascertain the fetal presentation (not usually of significance at this time) will reveal that approximately 1 in 3 fetuses present by the breech. Four weeks later the majority will have turned spontaneously so that at 34 weeks only 5% remain as malpresentations. Of this 5% most will have extended knees, a deviation from the normal attitude of complete flexion. The extended legs, by a splint-like action, make spontaneous version more difficult and may prevent it. This attitude is the cause of most breech presentations.

TYPES OF BREECH PRESENTATION

Four types of breech presentation are found (Figure 36).

(1)   Breech with extended legs. This, for the reasons stated, is the most common type of breech and is also known as the 'frank breech', the presenting part being the buttocks. The majority of breech presentations found in primigravidae are of this type.

(2)   The fully flexed breech, or complete breech, is found more commonly in multiparae when buttocks and feet present together.

(3)   Knee presentation (hips extended knees flexed).

(4)   Footling presentation (hips and knees extended).

Types (3) and (4) are uncommon.

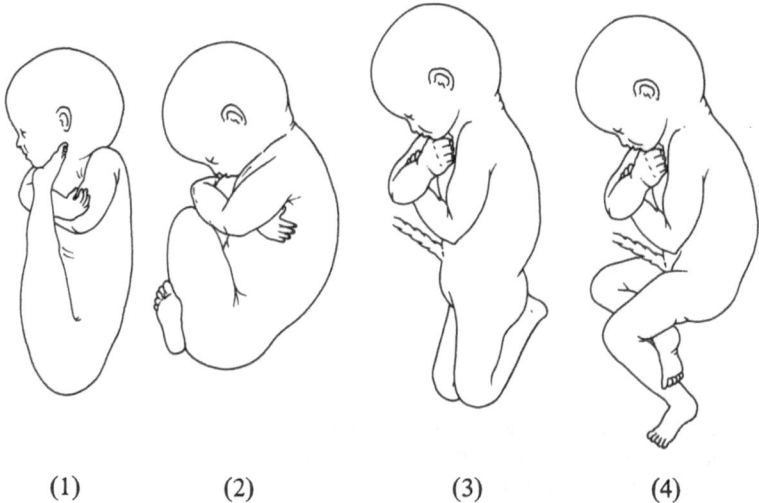

(1)   (2)   (3)   (4)

Figure 36   Types of breech presentation

DISADVANTAGES OF BREECH DELIVERY
These may be considered under two headings, maternal and fetal.

Maternal
Labour may be prolonged and thus carry with it increased risks of haemorrhage, shock and infection as well as possible psychological trauma. Furthermore, operative interference is more often necessary and soft tissue lacerations are more frequent although the free use of liberal episiotomy reduces this risk.

Fetal
The baby is at a greater risk of death or injury from two causes:

Intracranial haemorrhage. With a cephalic presentation, the head may be engaged for days or weeks before labour. Even when this is not so, the passage of the head through the pelvis is slow, especially when moulding is taking place. Delivery, too, in the second stage is usually well controlled. In a breech delivery the fetal head which has been situated in the uterine fundus for some time, must pass in and out of the bony pelvis within a few minutes or less. In these circumstances it is subject to a sudden compression force and often an even more quickly applied decompression which may lead to a tentorial tear and intracranial haemorrhage.

Asphyxia neonatorum. This may be due to

(1)   Cord prolapse which is an ever-present risk in all malpresentations. Furthermore, with a breech delivery the cord, which of course is visible as the fetal abdomen is born, is often compressed before the baby's mouth and nose are free.
(2)   Before delivery of the aftercoming head is accomplished but the rest of the baby is born, the partly emptied uterus may contract and retract on the placental site and impair the blood and oxygen supply to the fetus.

The dangers of (1) and (2) are considerably increased if there is any delay in the birth of the head.

The reported incidence of breech delivery varies and an average figure would be approximately 2%. There is little doubt, however, that perinatal mortality associated with this malpresentation is increased even when there are no other obstetric complications. The management remains controversial but the most important single factor in safe vaginal delivery of a breech at or near term is the practitioner's skill. So a specialist obstetrician should conduct the delivery.

Breech presentations, however, may be misdiagnosed or may have arisen shortly before the onset of labour, so all personnel who may be involved in maternity care should know how to cope in an emergency situation.

There is an increasing tendency to advocate routine caesarean section especially for preterm deliveries, and staffing and facilities available for antepartum investigations, monitoring in labour and care of the neonate may affect management. In addition to the experience of the practitioner other important factors include the estimated weight and maturity of the fetus, the type of breech (the frank breech with the baby's buttocks well applied to the cervix at the onset of labour is the most favourable) and the shape and size of the maternal pelvis. A routine lateral X-ray pelvimetry film should be taken, particularly if the patient is a primigravida. Caesarean section itself is associated with an increase in maternal morbidity (as well as mortality) and carries with it an increased risk of respiratory distress syndrome in the newborn. All these factors must be considered with care in each individual case, and the risks of abdominal and vaginal delivery to mother and baby compared. Elective caesarean section is preferable in primigravidae aged 35 years or more, or if there is any other obstetric complication such as contracted pelvis.

Some authorities may prefer to induce labour a week or so before term if all other circumstances appear satisfactory, and I often recommend this. I certainly prefer to avoid postmaturity where possible, because ossification of the fetal skull is progressive and the post-term skull is less able to mould with safety.

VERSION

In favourable circumstances the increased risk of breech delivery to mother and baby is small but attempts to correct the malpresentation prenatally are usually worthwhile. Turning the fetus around its longitudinal axis is known as *version*, and this may be either:

(1)   *External*, or via the abdominal wall performed before or during labour.
(2)   *Internal*, with a hand inside the uterus and when the cervix is fully dilated.
(3)   *Cephalic*, to make the head the presenting part.
(4)   *Podalic*, to turn the fetus into a breech presentation.

Internal version is always podalic, and in modern obstetrics is performed to extract the second twin found lying transversely.

External cephalic version

This procedure (Figure 37) is used to prevent breech delivery, but it should not be attempted before the 32nd or even the 34th week of pregnancy. If necessary, attempts may be repeated a few times at weekly intervals. Some obstetricians feel that if external cephalic version can be performed successfully, the baby would have turned itself spontaneously but this is contrary to my experience. Furthermore, I feel general anaesthesia for attempted version should not be used. There is a knack in performing external cephalic version and the breech should first be dislodged from the pelvis into the iliac fossa on the same side as the fetal back. Then the head is eased round towards the fetal abdomen (to maintain the attitude of flexion) until a transverse lie is achieved. At this stage the fetus will often slip spontaneously into a cephalic presentation when pressure is maintained, as shown in Figure 37(c).

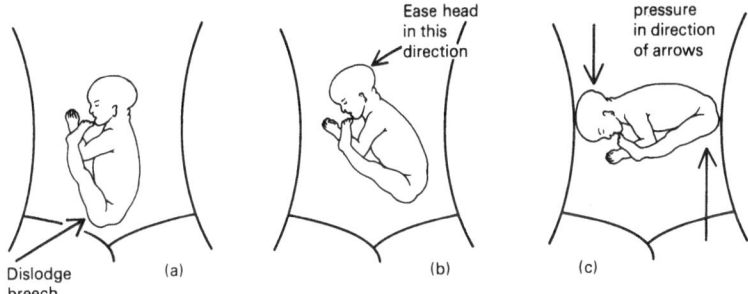

Figure 37 External cephalic version (a), (b) and (c)

The risks of performing external cephalic version are minimized by avoiding force. The risks involved are as follows.

(1) Premature labour may ensue.

(2) Placental separation with antepartum haemorrhage may occur, with an increased risk if the patient is hypertensive.

(3) Fetal–maternal haemorrhage is possible. Thus, if the patient has Rh-negative blood, version should be avoided or, if performed, an intramuscular injection of 100 mg of gammaglobulin is given.

(4) The cord may become entangled with the fetus or knots may be tied. The fetal heart slows after version attempts and must always be checked to ensure that normal rate and rhythm return within a few minutes.

In addition to hypertension mentioned above, contraindications to performing the manoeuvre include suspected multiple pregnancy or placenta praevia, and cases for elective caesarean section.

DIAGNOSIS OF BREECH PRESENTATION

The features that distinguish the head from the breech are that the former is hard, smooth, globular and mobile. The mobility is that of the head upon the neck and is still present when the fetal trunk is immobilized by an assistant applying pressure with the palms of both hands on the sides of the uterus. The breech at the fundus may give an impression of mobility by the entire fetus moving to and fro, but this will disappear if pressure is applied to the sides of the uterus as described. The groove between head and neck may be felt to aid correct diagnosis of presentation, but attempts to compare the sizes of the fetal poles are often misleading.

A woman with a breech presentation often complains of discomfort in the region of the fundus associated with pressure of the fetal head, and many patients feel more comfortable immediately after successful version and are able correctly to diagnose the presentation by their sensations. X-ray will indicate the presentation and on vaginal examination the sacrum, anus and buttocks and possibly feet are felt. It must be noted that on vaginal or rectal examination, the frank breech quite often feels hard, smooth and globular. The breech, however, does not have sutures and fontanelles, and the diagnosis of vertex presentation should not be made on vaginal examination unless one of these landmarks of the fetal skull is felt.

MECHANISM: LEFT SACRO-ANTERIOR POSITION

The mechanism of labour with the fetus in the left sacro-anterior position (LSA) is now described. The lie is longitudinal, the presentation podalic and the denominator is the sacrum which is entering the maternal pelvis opposite the left iliopectineal eminence (Figure 38).

The following steps take place:

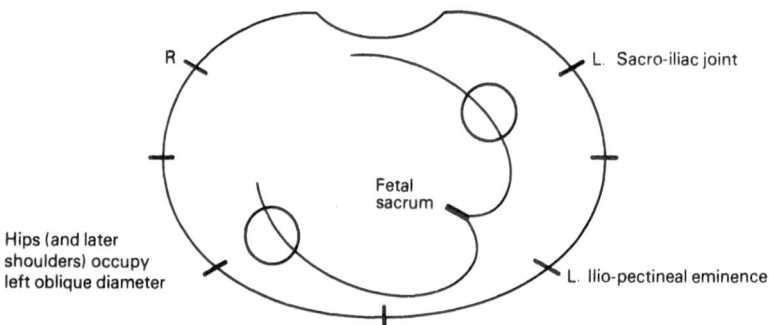

Figure 38   Breech in pelvic inlet in left sacro-anterior (LSA) position

(1)   Engagement. The bitrochanteric diameter (10 cm) engages in the left oblique diameter of the pelvis.

Note that the 'diameter' between the greater trochanters of the femora is greater than the diameter of engagement of the well-flexed head (suboccipito-bregmatic 9.5 cm), but the circumference of the breech is smaller. This fact is of practical importance as the breech may pass through a cervix which would not be fully dilated as far as the head is concerned. Bearing down efforts by the mother delivering a breech must not start too early.

(2)   With further descent, the anterior buttock rotates to the front (one-eighth of a circle) and appears below the pubic arch.

(3)   Lateral flexion of the spine occurs as the posterior buttock (or hip) sweeps over the perineum.

(4)   The shoulders enter the pelvic brim (in the left oblique diameter), the anterior one rotates to the front and appears below the symphysis followed by the posterior shoulder born posteriorly (in other words, internal rotation and birth of shoulders).

(5)   As internal rotation of the shoulders is taking place, the head enters the pelvis and flexes as it descends to the pelvic floor. Then internal rotation of the occiput to the front occurs and this shows itself as the back of the child rotates externally to the front.

(6)   The head is born by flexion. When the occipital protuberance is visible in the subpubic arch, the head may pivot out by flexion, as the chin, mouth and nose appear in that order over the perineum.

The management of the uncomplicated breech presentation
THE FIRST STAGE
The first stage of labour in any malpresentation tends to be prolonged. Therefore it becomes increasingly important to ensure that the patient is adequately hydrated, nourished and sedated as discussed above.

A further important factor to bear in mind when dealing with all malpresentations in which vaginal delivery is anticipated, is that there is a danger of premature rupture of the membranes and prolapse of the umbilical cord. The patient is thus kept in bed (which will also tend to prevent the mother bearing down too soon), and usually a vaginal examination is performed at the onset of labour and again when the membranes rupture. These examinations are conducted to ascertain the fetal presentation and position, and state of the cervix, and also to exclude presentation or prolapse of the cord. As placenta praevia is a possible cause of malpresentation, the obstetrician must be consulted before either a vaginal or rectal examination is attempted even in the absence of frank bleeding.

Enemata or suppositories are not generally administered. But in frank breech presentation in which the buttocks are well applied to the cervix, the risk of premature rupture of the membranes and prolapse of the cord is minimal. In such cases an enema may be given to avoid delay in labour associated with a loaded rectum. Otherwise management of the first stage in a breech presentation is as normal, but it is even more important to have everything ready for fetal resuscitation at delivery.

THE SECOND STAGE

Although all breech deliveries should be assisted, the principle to be observed in the absence of complications is one of minimal interference. The importance of ensuring that maternal bearing down efforts are not started too soon has been stated in describing the mechanism of labour (on previous page!). Preparations for delivery commence when the anterior buttock is well visible in the subpubic arch. The patient is then placed in the lithotomy position, skin cleansed and the area draped with sterile towels. Where possible, a one-piece sterile lithotomy sheet which entirely covers the lower limbs and abdomen is best. The bladder should be empty.

The accoucheur, suitably gowned, gloved and masked, should sit in front of the patient and observe the mechanism of labour in action – this sitting position enables the gloved hands to rest on the lap and the tendency to intervene unnecessarily is diminished! When the posterior buttock distends the perineum, a liberal episiotomy – certainly in all primigravidae – is performed as described on page 103). The episiotomy is performed at the height of a contraction, and if it is properly timed progress in delivery now becomes rapid. The baby's buttocks move upwards as there is lateral flexion of the spine which demonstrates well the curve of the birth canal. Occasionally, in a frank breech, the baby's feet require release from the vagina and this is achieved simply by hooking them out with a finger.

With the next contraction or two the fetus is born to the umbilicus. A loop of cord is gently eased down, palpated between index and ring fingers and displaced postero-laterally so that it lies in the hollow of the sacrum where it is less likely to be compressed. The pulsation in the cord indicates the action of the fetal heart. If at this stage it has become compressed there is still time, probably several minutes, in which to complete delivery. Thus it becomes almost an academic exercise to feel the cord; above all panic measures must be avoided. If the cord pulsation is strong and regular it is not compressed and there is no need for undue haste.

A sterile towel is now draped around the baby. This to some extent keeps the baby warm which prevents it gasping prematurely. The arms which are almost invariably flexed on the chest at the onset of labour, even when legs are extended, should be born spontaneously within the next few contractions. If necessary the attendant may free the baby's hands by hooking them out with a finger. If the arms are not born spontaneously they may be extended and assistance is essential. The attitude of the limbs may be ascertained by passing two fingers along the baby's abdomen. The arms, if flexed, will be felt on the baby's chest and may then be eased out by gentle traction on the hands. If, however, they are extended, the arms cannot be felt and the manoeuvre described below is performed.

The back of the child which was facing laterally will be seen to rotate to the front as internal rotation of the occiput occurs ((5), page 111). Maternal efforts to deliver the baby's head once it has passed completely into the true pelvis are of little use. Yet the head, to be born by flexion, must pass so deeply into the pelvis that the occipital protuberance becomes visible below the pubis. The head may be ready for delivery when the baby's hairline is seen, but the occipital protuberance should be felt. The *Burns—Marshall* manoeuvre is now employed for delivery. The baby is allowed to hang down for a minute or so while suprapubic pressure is applied with one hand. The forces used to enable the head to descend for delivery are thus the baby's body weight plus that of the suprapubic pressure, and this procedure ensures that the head remains flexed.

When the occipital protuberance is born, the manoeuvre is completed by carrying the fetus by its feet in an arc upward and over towards the mother's abdomen. This enables the head to pivot out by flexion as described in mechanism (6) (Figures 39 (a) and (b)). The baby's chin, mouth and nose will appear in order over the perineum at which point all movement ceases while the baby's air passages are cleared. The delivery of the baby's head is then completed slowly.

The important points to remember when conducting an uncomplicated breech delivery are:

(1)   Do not rush the maternal bearing-down efforts before ensuring that the cervix is fully dilated.
(2)   Perform a liberal episiotomy.
(3)   Do not apply traction to the fetus unless completely able to cope with extended arms.
(4)   When the Burns—Marshall manoeuvre is used, do not:
   (a)   apply suprapubic pressure too energetically,
   (b)   pull the fetus upwards by its feet too soon, as the head will not deliver unless it is able to pivot out by flexion as described.

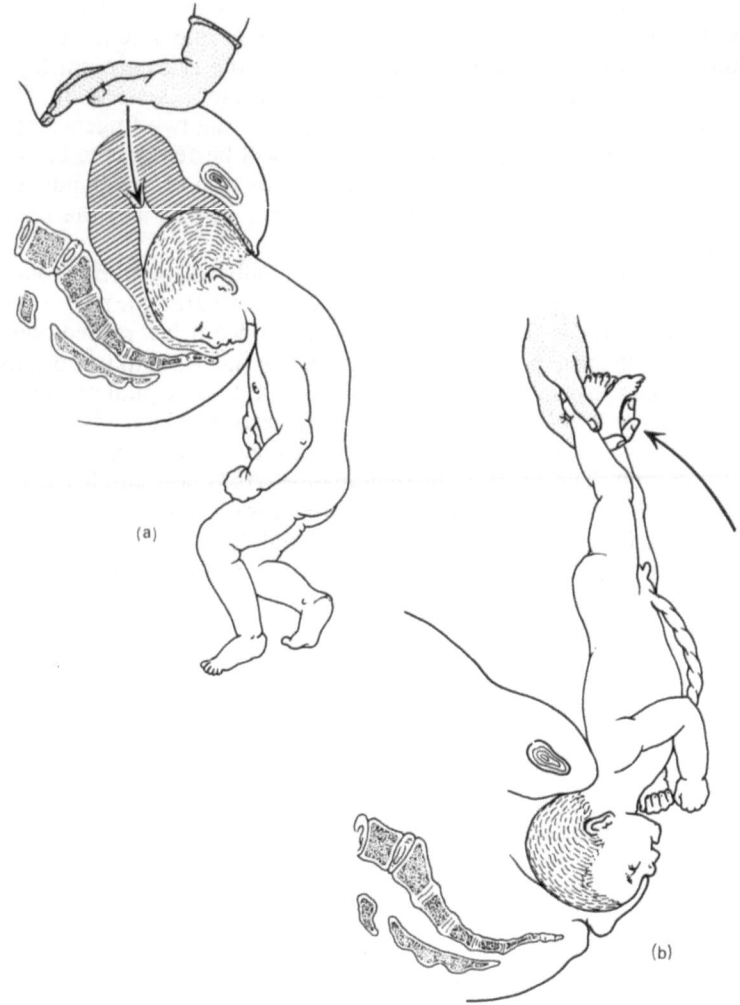

Figure 39   The Burns–Marshall manoeuvre: (a) baby hangs down and suprapubic pressure is applied, (b) when occipital protuberance is born
the baby is carried by its feet in an arc as shown

If there is delay in delivery of the aftercoming head it is possible to
allow air into the vagina for the fetus by retracting the perineum digitally or with the aid of a speculum, but it is an act of despair which puts
the life of the fetus in jeopardy. Other methods of delivery of the
aftercoming head are described below.

Management of the complicated breech delivery

There are several causes for delay in the birth of the buttocks, shoulders and/or the aftercoming head in breech deliveries. These include poor uterine muscle action, or the baby may be too big or the pelvis too small. Possible disproportion or other obstetric complications might indicate the need for elective caesarean section. However, delay in delivery may be due to causes applicable only to breech deliveries and are associated with the attitude of extension. Management of these complications is discussed below.

DELAY IN THE BIRTH OF THE BUTTOCKS

Decades ago extended legs in a breech were believed to act as a splint to the fetal spine thereby preventing lateral flexion and spontaneous delivery. Thus, breech extraction under general anaesthesia was the accepted mode of delivery. From earlier discussion it will be seen that the attitude of extended legs is the most common cause for breech presentation, and the old idea of a splinting action was usually wrong – usually, but not always. If there is delay in the birth of the buttocks, groin traction with a finger may be applied, where the finger is hooked around the fetal groin (preferably the anterior one) and traction applied in a downward direction. Similar traction may be applied to the posterior groin if it can be reached with ease. Traction must be applied only during a uterine contraction and analgesia is necessary.

It is desirable for all patients undergoing breech delivery to be given a pudendal nerve block at the start of the second stage. If this is not possible the perineum may be infiltrated with 0.5% lignocaine. Traction applied to deliver the buttocks and legs will often cause the arms to extend as they are caught up while the baby is being pulled downwards. Extended arms may not provide a problem to an experienced obstetrician conducting a breech delivery in a properly equipped unit, but should be prevented where possible by avoiding traction.

Older methods of breech extraction by 'pulling down a leg' required general anaesthesia. Traction to limbs must be applied distally to ankle or wrist and never to thigh or upper arm. In extracting a frank breech under general anaesthesia, the obstetrician reached the foot by flexing the knee with pressure exerted by two fingers in the popliteal fossa and then passing the fingers to the ankle. To reach the hands of extended arms, the accessible posterior arm was flexed by pushing it over the baby's face (rather like a cat washing its face after licking its paw). If the anterior arm was so tightly lodged under the pubis that it could not be delivered, the fetus was rotated manually through 180° by gripping its pelvis and turning it so that its face turned towards the extended arm. The latter often flexed during this rotation, but if not there was more room available in the hollow of the sacrum. (If the reader stretches an arm above the head and then faces it, the flexion action will be demonstrated. If the face is turned away from the arm, there is a tendency for the arm to be displaced behind the neck; this would be more difficult to deliver.)

DELAY IN THE BIRTH OF THE SHOULDERS
This is usually due to extended arms and is best dealt with by using the *Lövset manoeuvre* in which the arms are flexed by rotating the fetus externally using the pelvic grip. This rotation is performed when the posterior arm is in the pelvis below the sacral promontory, and this is usually found when the lower angle of the anterior scapula is just visible. The fetus is rotated through 180° to place the posterior arm directly anteriorly. The arm will flex and may be delivered by hooking out gently with a finger around the baby's wrist. Gentle traction is applied to the fetus during the rotatory movement. The fetus is then rotated in the opposite direction during which the remaining arm is flexed and may be delivered. Pudendal nerve block provides adequate analgesia for this manoeuvre.

DELAY IN THE BIRTH OF THE HEAD
The importance of ensuring that the breech has not passed through an incompletely dilated cervix must again be stressed. Backward rotation of the occiput rarely occurs and commonly delay is associated with some extension of the head which has not passed low enough in the pelvis to be born by flexion. The methods of dealing with this are as follows.

The Burns—Marshall manoeuvre
As described above this flexes the head. If delivery cannot be achieved the midwife uses jaw and shoulder traction.

Jaw and shoulder traction
Also called the *Mauriceau—Smellie—Veit manoeuvre* this is really one of jaw flexion and shoulder traction. The fetus is made to straddle the right forearm the elbow of which is depressed (Figure 40). One finger is inserted into the baby's mouth and two others are placed on each side of the jaw or maxilla. Gentle traction will flex the head. The other hand is placed over the baby's shoulders and round its neck so that a fingertip rests on each of the baby's sternoclavicular joints. It is important to ensure that the fingertips rest squarely on the joints so traction may be applied without causing damage. (Students may like to palpate their own joints which are obvious prominences and to practise the manoeuvre on a model fetus.) A third finger exerting pres-

sure below the occiput may also be used to promote flexion. *Traction* is first applied downwards and backwards and after the occipital protuberance is born, the upward curving arc of the birth canal is followed.

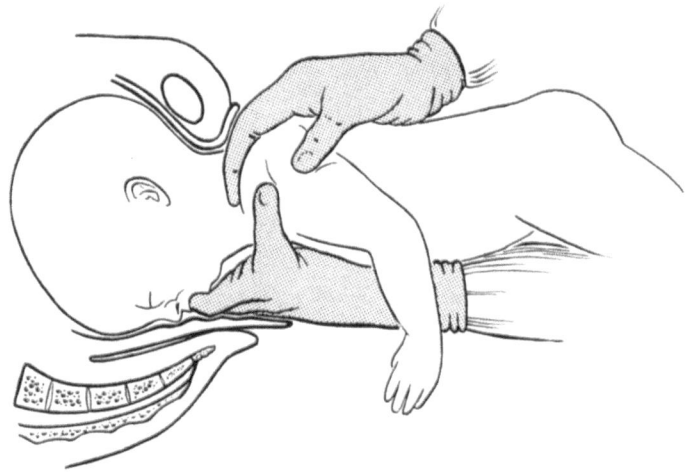

Figure 40 The Mauriceau–Smellie–Veit manoeuvre

Forceps extraction
This provides the best method of controlled delivery of the aftercoming head if there is any delay, and especially when pudendal nerve block has been given. An assistant supports the fetus while the obstetrician gently slips the blades of the forceps beneath it (Figure 41).

CAESAREAN SECTION
The role of elective abdominal delivery for breech presentation has been discussed. If there is any delay in the first stage of labour a careful reassessment of all factors should be made before deciding on the best mode of delivery. This, too, is sometimes necessary even in the second stage when the breech remains high in the pelvis. Caesarean section cannot possibly save a baby if there is delay after it has been partially delivered vaginally!

FETAL HOLDS
There are only three parts of the fetus that the accoucheur may hold or grip for purposes of applying traction or rotation without causing damage. These are:

(1) The baby's feet which may be held to apply traction on the breech.

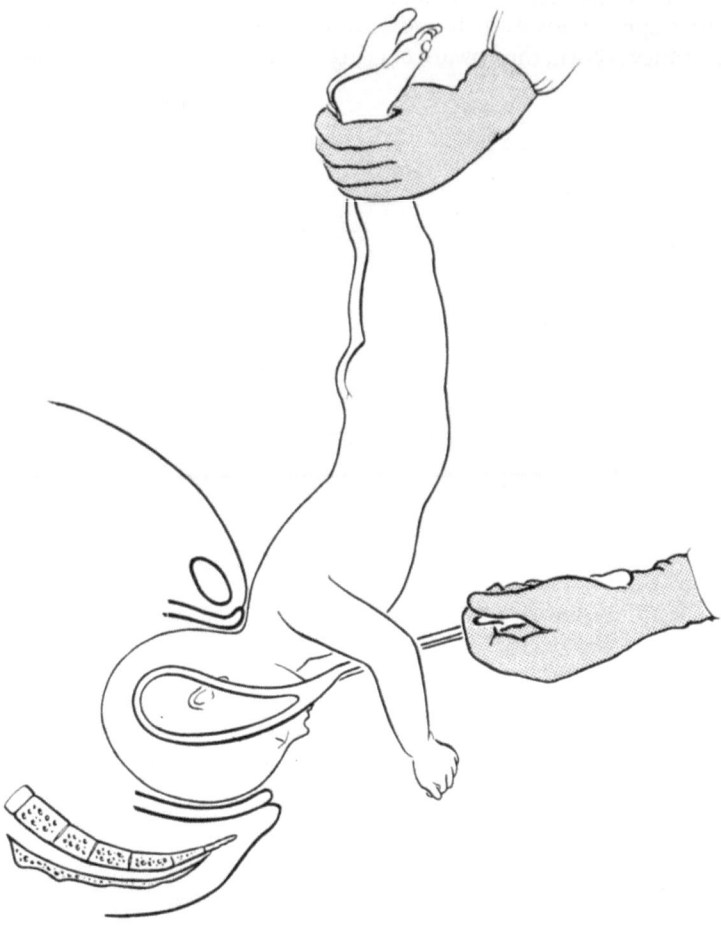

Figure 41 Forceps application to aftercoming head

(2)   The pelvic grip − used for performing the Lövset manoeuvre. In this the thumbs rest on the fetal sacrum and the index fingers on the pubic bones.
(3)   The sternoclavicular joints, upon which the fingertips rest to apply shoulder traction to deliver the aftercoming head in a breech delivery.

The midwife must always take great care to ensure that the baby's abdomen is not gripped or held.

11

Face, brow and shoulder presentations

If the head presents and adopts an attitude of full extension, the result is a face presentation. The majority of these cases are not due to the causes as listed for malpresentation in general (Chapter 10) but are associated with an excessive tone of the extensor muscles of the fetus (muscles passing from the fetal spine to the head). Full extension may have taken place during labour which had commenced with the head of the fetus badly flexed in an occipito-posterior position or partially extended as a brow presentation. This is *secondary* face presentation which is more common than *primary* — that is, a fully extended cephalic presentation before the onset of labour. The incidence of face delivery is approximately 1 in 500.

Face presentation
MECHANISM
The mechanism of a face presentation is analogous to that of an occipito-anterior position except for that fact that the head is born by flexion. The denominator is the *mentum* or point of the chin and the diameter of engagement is the submento-bregmatic (9.5 cm), the same measurement as that of the engaging diameter of the fully flexed vertex (suboccipito-bregmatic), so usually face delivery presents no problems. As descent occurs, the chin (which in the left mento-anterior or LMA position enters the pelvis in the right oblique diameter) usually rotates to the front and emerges from beneath the symphysis. The head is born by flexion; restitution and internal rotation, and birth of shoulders and trunk follow as described for vertex mechanisms (page 88).

There is, however, one other important feature of face presentation which differs from that of the vertex. In a small number of cases the chin may rotate posteriorly to the hollow of the sacrum. When this *persistent mento-posterior* position occurs, normal delivery is impossible as the head and chest of the baby are attempting to enter the pel-

119

vis together. The persistent occipito-posterior position can deliver spontaneously face-to-pubis, but the mento-posterior position must be corrected either by rotation with forceps or manually, or delivered by caesarean section. Flexion to a vertex presentation is possible, but excessive extensor muscle tone may make this difficult.

DIAGNOSIS
Face presentation may be considered likely when on abdominal palpation a deep groove is felt between the back of the baby and its head, and the prominence of the latter on the ventral surface of the fetus is absent. The fetal heart is best heard over its chest. X-ray may indicate the attitude of extension. The diagnosis is usually made on vaginal examination in early labour when the irregularities of eyes, nose, mouth and chin may be felt. If on vaginal examination an orifice is found, the examiner should consider the question of whether the orifice is mouth or anus − this will diminish the likelihood of confusing breech with face presentations.

PRACTICAL POINTS IN MANAGEMENT
If the chin rotates anteriorly vaginal delivery is usually achieved without undue difficulty. Digital pressure under the chin may help to keep the head fully extended until the chin escapes below the pubis and the head can be born by flexion.

The pressure on the soft tissues of the fetal face during labour will usually result in gross oedema of eyelids and lips making the baby appear quite monstrous on delivery; but the swellings disappear entirely within 48 hours. It is therefore of the utmost importance to inform both parents before delivery occurs that, as a result of the baby coming face first, these swellings will probably be present but that they are transitory.

Brow presentation
Brow presentation is a cephalic presentation in which the head is extended but only partially so. The causes for this and the possible diagnosis by abdominal palpation are similar to those discussed above for face presentations. The positive diagnosis of brow presentation is normally made in labour when on vaginal examination the supraorbital ridges and anterior fontanelle are felt. The skull diameter attempting to engage is the *mento-vertical*, which is that extending from the point of the chin to the furthest point on the vault of the skull. The measurement normally exceeds 13 cm so that the head cannot engage, and a mechanism for vaginal delivery as a brow is impossible. A brow presentation must, therefore, be either flexed into a vertex,

extended into a face or delivered by caesarean section. I prefer abdominal delivery if manual extension of the head would lead to a mento-posterior position. Flexion to a vertex is often difficult especially as the aetiological factor may be high tone of the extensor muscles.

If extension of the head is associated with gross fetal abnormality each case must be individually evaluated. The particular abnormality, facilities available, experience of the obstetrician, and the patient herself as well as the conditions in which her next confinement may take place, must all be taken into consideration. Most obstetricians in the United Kingdom, practising under good conditions, consider caesarean section safer for the mother than destructive operations on the abnormal fetus.

Shoulder presentation: transverse and oblique lie
DIAGNOSIS
A transverse or oblique lie is diagnosed by abdominal palpation when both poles of the fetus are found to be out of alignment with the long-itudinal axis of the uterus. An oblique lie is often easier to diagnose than a breech presentation in which the head may be tucked away behind the costal margin. When an unstable fetal presentation is found in the last 6 weeks of pregnancy the following points must be considered.

Exclusion of all possible causes
After excluding all possible causes for the malpresentation, consider especially the possibility of a developmental abnormality of the uterus. Much of the female genital tract develops from two columns of cells found on either side of the fetal abdominal cavity. These form two ducts, the *Müllerian ducts*, which normally come together in the midline and after fusing, the septum between the two ducts is absorbed (Figure 42). Congenital abnormalities that may occur include vary-

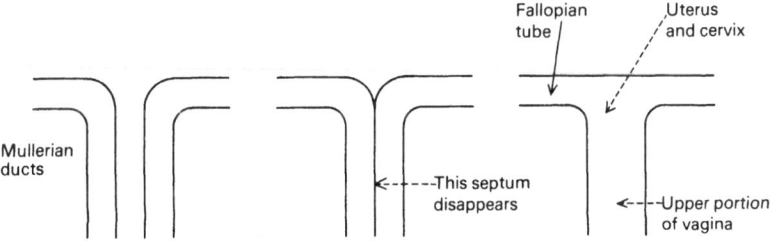

Figure 42   Schematic representation and development of the genital tract

ing degrees of failure of fusion of the Müllerian ducts. A minor malformation may be associated with a small dip in the uterine fundus (*arcuate uterus*) and in extreme degrees there may be two separate genital tracts. Major congenital abnormalities are associated with subfertility or cause abortion, and minor degrees, which are not uncommon, predispose to unstable fetal lie.

As genital and urinary tracts have developmental connections it is important to investigate fully the kidneys and ureter after a pregnancy associated with a congenital abnormality of the uterus has ended. Intravenous pyelography may reveal further anomalies.

Antepartum management
The occurrence of labour with the fetus lying transversely or obliquely may be prevented by external cephalic version (see page 109). Pads and binders are occasionally applied to the abdomen after successful version but on the whole they tend to be ineffective. Although applied very firmly to maintain a longitudinal fetal lie, binders rapidly work loose especially in an ambulant patient. An unstable lie in a multiparous patient may correct itself as term approaches, but the risk of premature rupture of the membranes and prolapse of the cord is always present. Therefore, it is often advisable for the patient to be admitted to hospital 1 or 2 weeks preterm so that she is under constant supervision while awaiting the onset of labour.

If the pregnancy is approaching full term, and the cervix is effaced and 2 cm or more dilated, the obstetrician may consider artificial rupture of the forewaters after successful external cephalic version. As the liquor drains away, the practitioner should not remove the fingers from the vagina but ensure that the fetal head enters the pelvis with no evidence of the cord. The patient thereafter remains propped-up in bed, and in these conditions abdominal pads and binders are occasionally of value. Continuous fetal heart monitoring is advisable, but if there are no facilities for this, very frequent recordings must be made. There is the risk of an oblique lie recurring with prolapsed cord so it is essential to be prepared for immediate ceasarean section.

Management in labour
If the transverse or oblique lie is first diagnosed when the patient is in labour the treatment is either as above or, if version cannot be successfully performed, immediate caesarean section is indicated. If the cervix is fully dilated and the fetus (usually the second twin) is lying transversely, treatment consists of internal podalic version followed by breech extraction as described in Chapter 10.

If the condition of transverse or oblique lie remains undiagnosed and untreated in labour, the latter will be obstructed and the uterus will rupture.

12

The umbilical cord:
presentation and prolapse

There is a wide variation of length of the umbilical cord at term so that any measurement between 40 and 75 cm may be regarded as normal. The cord, the connecting link between fetus and placenta, usually contains two arteries and one vein which lie in a mucoid connective tissue or *Wharton's jelly*. The arteries, which carry oxygen and nutrients to the fetus, have a strong muscle coat and are formed by the union of the vessels seen coursing over the fetal surface of the placenta. These in their turn are formed by the fusion of the small vessels of the chorionic villi. The single vein of the cord arises from the umbilical vein and transports carbon dioxide and other waste products to the placenta where they pass into the maternal bloodstream and are excreted. In about 1% of umbilical cords only one artery may be present. Although fetal growth is not affected by the absence of the second artery, the anomaly may be associated with a fetal abnormality and it is more commonly present in twin pregnancies and premature deliveries.

An uninterrupted and free flow of blood through the vessels of the cord is essential for adequate oxygenation of the fetus and if this flow is obstructed before the baby can breathe air or oxygen, action without delay is necessary if the fetus is to survive.

Abnormalities of the cord
The more important abnormalities of the cord are knots, fetal entanglement with the cord, and unusual length.

KNOTS
The cord blood vessels, and especially the vein, are longer than the cord itself and they thus tend to become twisted and form loops. *True knots* in the cord are uncommon and the life of the fetus would be in jeopardy only if the loops were pulled together tightly. *False knots* are of no clinical significance and are nodular projections of the cord

associated with thickened collections of Wharton's jelly and varicosities of the vessels.

FETAL ENTANGLEMENT WITH THE CORD
The cord may wind itself around the neck of the fetus or loop itself around the limbs. Sometimes intrauterine movements, but more often fetal descent during labour, may tighten the loops and cause anoxia as the cord vessels are constricted.

UNUSUAL LENGTH
A very short cord may cause delay in delivery, placental separation, or the cord may rupture. Herniae into the cord occur, and cases are reported in which the cord was totally absent and the fetus attached to the placenta through a hernia. These are all rare accidents. An abnormally long cord is more likely to prolapse or entangle with the fetus.

Presentation and prolapse
The presenting part, by definition, is that part which lies over the internal os of the cervix and is normally an area of the vertex. If, however, a loop of cord lies before the baby and over the internal os, the cord is said to be presenting as long as the forewaters remain intact. *Presentation* of the cord becomes *prolapse* immediately the forewaters rupture. If the cord has passed through the cervix into the vagina or its presence is first detected when it is seen protruding from the vulva (not uncommon) then 'prolapse' is obviously established, but the distinction between presentation and prolapse of the cord depends on whether the membranes of the forewaters are intact or have ruptured. The distinction is clinically important because the fetal condition is usually satisfactory while the membranes remain intact, but the cord may well become compressed as soon as they rupture. Compression of the cord between the fetus and the bony pelvis or cervix will cause anoxia and fetal death unless rapid action is taken.

PREDISPOSING CAUSES
Malpresentations and causes for malpresentations (Chapter 10) must all be considered. Indeed, every time a vaginal examination is performed in labour, the practitioner considers the possibility of presentation or prolapse of the cord, especially if the vertex is not closely applied to the lower segment of the uterus at the onset of labour. Other predisposing causes include unusual length of the cord, and manoeuvres such as version and manual rotation of the fetus.

DIAGNOSIS
This is made on vaginal examination or visually when during labour
the membranes rupture spontaneously and the cord protrudes from
the introitus. This may happen in a multipara in whom the fetal head
was found to be entering the pelvis at the start of labour. The other
features that point to the diagnosis are those of fetal distress (page
95), and it is important to remember that the rate and regularity of
pulsation in the cord is that of the fetal heart. The cord, which is felt
between the index and middle finger, is easily recognizable if prolapsed. However, when presenting in a tense bag of forewaters, it may
be difficult to define a cord-like structure and pulsation only will be
detected. It is not uncommon to feel pulsation in the vaginal fornices
on deep penetration during vaginal examination in labour and this
sometimes causes unnecessary concern. The uterine arteries have cervical and vaginal branches and the latter anastomose with the vaginal
arteries. The examiner, especially one with long fingers, may appreciate pulsation from a maternal blood vessel. There should be no difficulty in distinguishing maternal pulsation from that in the umbilical
cord. If pulsation is at the same rate as the maternal pulse it is due to a
maternal blood vessel, and if the rate is that of the fetal heart,
presentation of the cord is diagnosed. The latter can also be diagnosed
by ultrasonic echogram.

TREATMENT
The conditions necessitate urgent treatment and it is assumed that the
pregnancy has reached a stage of maturity in which the fetus is viable.
The management is as follows.

Presentation of the cord
Caesarean section should be performed without delay. While preparations for this procedure are in hand the membranes must be kept intact for as long as possible. Thus the patient is kept in bed the foot of
which is raised to a degree consistent with her comfort (*the Trendelenburg position*). The fetal condition is best monitored continuously and
all attendants must be prepared to deal with prolapse of the cord at
any stage.

Prolapse of the cord
The cord is first palpated. If pulsation is totally absent and the fetus is
dead, no treatment is indicated for the condition of prolapsed cord,
but the underlying cause may require correction. So if, for example,
the fetal lie is transverse appropriate measures are necessary to ensure
that the mother's life is not at risk from obstructed labour. If, on the
other hand, a loop of cord prolapsed and the fetal head followed with

no evidence of disproportion, no active measures are indicated if the fetus has failed to survive. The mother, however, will require the greatest degree of support, and possibly additional sedation.

If pulsation in the cord is present, whether strong and regular, or feeble, rapid, irregular and/or slow, or it is believed that the fetus can survive — in other words no pulsation is felt but the fetal heart was present just prior to the accident, the treatment is best summed up as: *deliver the baby immediately or keep the pressure off the cord until immediate delivery is possible.*

Immediate delivery can be achieved by either caesarean section, or if the second stage of labour has been reached by forceps or breech extraction. Occasionally, if the head is distending the perineum, a liberal episiotomy may suffice.

The best method of *keeping the pressure off the cord* is to make the patient adopt the *knee–elbow position* (or knee–chest position) with her buttocks as high in the air as is possible. This posture will make the presenting part move out of the pelvis and relieve pressure on the cord. If, however, a loop of cord has prolapsed out of the vulva, it should be eased back into the vagina and/or wrapped in sterile gauze soaked in warm saline to prevent spasm of the blood vessels which may occur due to hypothermia. The patient is kept in this posture until all preparations are ready for delivery. This often means transference to the operating table for abdominal delivery. The patient should be moved maintaining the knee–elbow position on the stretcher or trolley until placed on the operating table in the Trendelenburg position.

A cord may prolapse unexpectedly in a multigravida who is having strong contractions every few minutes and in whom the cervix is still less than half dilated. The baby's head may have been entering the pelvis and progress was apparently satisfactory until the membranes ruptured and the cord became visible. Although it may not be the most comfortable attitude, the knee–elbow position of the mother has saved the lives of countless babies. Constant reassurance to the mother is of utmost importance.

The other method of relieving pressure on the cord is to insert a hand into the vagina and push the presenting part upward. Pure oxygen administered to the mother is also useful.

Attempts to replace the cord and make the presenting part engage by methods such as sitting the patient up and applying abdominal pads and binders are generally useless. It is conceivable that a small knuckle of cord felt alongside the head may be replaced digitally if no other facilities for treatment are at hand.

13

Twins and multiple pregnancy

The average incidence of twin pregnancy is approximately 1 in 80 although the figure shows a wide variation geographically and is greater in older patients and those with a family history of multiple pregnancy. The variation is due to the differing incidence of *binovular* (*non-identical* or *dizygous*) twins in which two mature ova are shed and fertilized at the same time. Both ova may arise from one Graafian follicle or, less commonly, two follicles maturate in 1 month. The incidence of *uniovular* (*identical* or *monozygous*) twins appears to be more constant, but the reason for this is not clear. In this type only one ovum is fertilized and the resultant zygote divides into two blasto-meres which separate and develop individually. The early blastomeres are totipotent − in other words, each is capable of developing into a complete organism and twinning may occur at various stages in the initial cell divisions. Uniovular twins are always of the same sex. Careful examination of the placenta and membranes may reveal the type of twins born, although, in view of the different stages at which twinning is possible, this is not always the case.

Each of binovular twins (which may or may not be of the same sex) has its own placenta, chorion and amnion. Although the substance of the two placentae may be fused, each has its own circulation and the septum between the two fetal sacs consists of double layers of amnion and chorion. Identical twins share one placenta with one chorion and two amniotic sacs, so that the septum contains no chorionic tissue and consists of two layers of thin transparent amnion only. A big differ-ence in birthweight is found more commonly in uniovular twins as they compete with each other for the shared placenta. Their blood groups and tissue typing are identical.

The incidence of triplets is about 1 in 8000 and they are generally due to the fact that two or three ova are shed and fertilized concur-rently. If two ova only are involved the triplets must contain one pair of uniovular twins. Higher numbers of babies born after individual pregnancy are being increasingly reported today due to an increased use of fertility drugs. Chorionic gonadotrophin and ovarian stimulants such as clomiphene are of value in selected cases of subfertility, but multiple pregnancies are more likely when they are given to a woman who is already ovulating.

Most, if not all experienced practitioners, have at times missed diagnosing a twin pregnancy. It appears to some that to diagnose twins in the presence of a singleton pregnancy is preferable to making the error in the other direction. This may be understandable but patients can become quite distressed over uncertainty engendered by a remark made even lightheartedly that there may possibly be more than one fetus present. So if there is any uncertainty, the examiner must ensure that steps are taken to establish a correct diagnosis at the earliest opportunity.

Diagnosis of multiple pregnancy

Features of importance in making and establishing a diagnosis of twins are:

(1) *Personal and/or family history* of multiple pregnancy.

(2) *Pelvic and abdominal examination.* The uterus may be larger than anticipated from the menstrual history at the initial pelvic examination and before the 12th week. Later in pregnancy abdominal palpation may show that size and increase in size are excessive, especially if hydramnios is present. Acute hydramnios in one fetal sac of uniovular twins is no rarity when a fluid thrill may be elicited to indicate this. In the second half of pregnancy three or more fetal poles (head or breech) can be felt, and limbs seem more numerous.

(3) *Ultrasonic echogram.* Twin pregnancy may be demonstrable before the 8th week by showing the presence of two heads or two fetal sacs.

(4) *Fetal hearts.* Two fetal hearts beating can be demonstrated by ultrascan at an early stage. The counting of separate fetal hearts by stethoscope must be performed simultaneously by two observers and the difference in rate must be wide enough to allow for human error before diagnosing twins on this account.

(5) *X-ray* is best deferred until after the 30th week of pregnancy. Repeat ultrascan is preferable before this time.

(6) *Complications* of pregnancy more frequently found in twin pregnancies are:

    (a)   Nausea and vomiting in the early months.

(b) Pressure symptoms, especially in the last trimester, are more marked and include varicose veins, haemorrhoids, oedema of legs, heartburn and abdominal discomfort.
(c) Hydramnios, which also increases the severity of pressure effects.
(d) Anaemia.
(e) Pre-eclampsia.
(f) Premature onset of labour.

Management of multiple pregnancy

The importance of prenatal supervision must be stressed and frequency of examinations often needs to be increased in the second half of pregnancy. Dietetic principles are as normal and adequate rest is essential. Constant watch for anaemia associated with both iron and folic acid deficiencies must be maintained. As mentioned earlier (page 57) there is an increased demand for folic acid because this substance is necessary for the production of DNA to ensure normal cell division. The demand is met by all patients taking an additional 5 mg daily in the second half of pregnancy.

In view of the increased risks of pre-eclampsia developing in the latter months, and of premature labour resulting in even smaller babies, it has been the practice in many centres to advise hospitalization for a month during the critical period from 30 to 34 weeks. Bed-rest will diminish the need to recommend induction of labour on account of pre-eclampsia and increase the blood supply to the placenta, the efficiency of which should be monitored in the last 2 months of pregnancy. Whether hospitalization is necessary in the absence of complications is debatable and depends upon the circumstances of the individual patient. I do not institutionalize patients routinely provided that they are able to ensure adequate rest in the knowledge that admission can be arranged at any time if required.

Induction of labour may be indicated for increasingly severe pre-eclampsia, hydramnios, diminishing placental efficiency, and occasionally to alleviate severe discomfort associated with overstretching of the muscles. Adequate fetal maturity and the optimum time for delivery may be assessed (page 190).

Management of labour in multiple pregnancy

THE FIRST STAGE

This may be prolonged, and is managed on lines similar to those for malpresentations (see Chapter 10). Preparations are made to receive two premature infants even if full term has been reached, so the paediatrician with access to two incubators should be available.

THE SECOND STAGE

The first twin is usually delivered normally provided the fetal lie is longitudinal and no other obstetric complications are present. An episiotomy is indicated in almost all deliveries in the interests of the babies. The cord is very firmly ligatured or clamped before it is cut, as bleeding from the placental end may involve loss from the twin *in utero*.

When the first baby is delivered, the lie of the second twin is determined by abdominal palpation and if necessary external version is performed to make this longitudinal. When the presentation is considered to be either cephalic or podalic a vaginal examination is performed to check this. If the uterus is still contracting the forewaters are ruptured and the fingers remain in the vagina as liquor escapes to ensure that head or breech descends without cord prolapse. There is no need for haste to rupture the membranes which is not performed if the uterus is inactive or there is doubt as to the presenting part. But on the other hand it is nevertheless most undesirable for the mother to have to wait for hours (or even days!) to elapse before delivery of the second twin. It should also be noted that the lie and presentation of the second twin is of no significance until after the first baby is delivered.

If the lie of the second twin cannot be satisfactorily corrected and remains transverse or oblique, treatment usually consists of internal podalic version, achieved by the obstetrician identifying and pulling down a foot, followed by breech extraction. General anaesthesia for this manoeuvre is desirable.

Forceps extraction of the second twin may be indicated to hasten delivery in the event of fetal distress or failure to progress. Caesarean section to deliver a second twin is rarely necessary provided the cervix remains fully dilated and the practitioner is experienced.

THE THIRD STAGE

In twin pregnancies the myometrium has been overstretched, labour tends to be longer and the placental area is larger than with a singleton pregnancy. The patient is thus more likely to sustain a postpartum haemorrhage. Otherwise the third stage is managed normally. An oxytocic injection is given after the birth of the anterior shoulder of the second twin (if a cephalic presentation) but only if there is no possibility of a further fetus *in utero*.

Rare conditions

Conditions of particular interest are: *locked twins*: 'locking' occurs in various degrees. Full locking takes place when the first twin, a breech presentation, has delivered vaginally to the level of the neck and the head of the second twin enters the pelvis. The first baby's neck is stretched as its head is forced out of the pelvis into the abdomen. The head of the second baby must be manually displaced out of the pelvis before effecting delivery if destructive operations are to be avoided.

'Twinning' of the uniovular types as mentioned above may take place at various stages of development. It may occur after the formation of the amniotic sac (uniamniotic twins) or later still when conjoined twins may result.

14

Pre-eclampsia

The term 'toxaemias of pregnancy' was originally used to include a heterogeneous collection of conditions, all of which had an obscure aetiology. Thus included under this heading were various skin rashes, hyperemesis, polyneuritis and ptyalism (excessive salivation) of pregnancy. Today the term 'toxaemia' is used by most authorities to include the states of pre-eclampsia, essential hypertension and the chronic nephritis group of illnesses (for the latter see page 63).

The word 'toxaemia', so entrenched in the minds of doctors and midwives, is in itself a misnomer, because although the aetiology of the condition remains obscure and complex, a toxin as such is unlikely to be the responsible agent.

Definition of pre-eclampsia

Pre-eclampsia may be defined as a condition peculiar to pregnant women which, if unchecked, can lead to eclampsia and its associated epileptiform convulsions. The condition is of considerable importance because it is one of the commonest complications of pregnancy (second only to anaemia) in the United Kingdom and plays a major role in both maternal and perinatal mortality and morbidity. The reported incidence varies widely from less than 5% to about 15% as the criteria for making the diagnosis differ. It is, however, safer to regard even minor degrees of hypertension not uncommonly seen in the latter weeks of pregnancy (*pregnancy-induced hypertension*, or *PIH*) as a manifestation of pre-eclampsia, and by including these cases the 15% figure seems more accurate.

Pre-eclampsia may not only lead to eclampsia, but may also be associated with accidental antepartum haemorrhage (abruptio placentae). The number of maternal deaths in the United Kingdom from these conditions has declined progressively over the past decades (from 246 per 100 000 population in 1952—54, to 39 in 1973—75), but the triennial reports on *Confidential Enquiries into Maternal Deaths in*

England and Wales published by the Department of Health and Social Security shows the 'avoidable factor' incidence has not been so diminished. Patient, general practitioner and consultant figure quite prominently in the groups held to be responsible for the avoidable factors. The vital importance of ensuring that adequate prenatal care is given to all mothers is thus underlined.

Aetiology of pre-eclampsia

Before the clinical aspects of pre-eclampsia are considered, a brief survey of a few of the many theories about its aetiology is of interest. Any theory proposed should explain some, if not all, of the clinical features of the condition. Thus, pre-eclampsia occurs in all gravida groups, the highest rate being found in primigravidae. It generally occurs in the last months of pregnancy and usually, but not always, clears up after delivery. The complication is more common in association with twins and diabetes mellitus, and it is encountered in early pregnancy if hydatidiform mole (see Chapter 17) is present.

It is not surprising that researchers have turned their attention to the placenta and its hormones and metabolism. The primigravida is experiencing the hormone changes for the first time, with the placenta elaborating large quantities of oestrogens and progestogens and fluctuating amounts of chorionic gonadotrophin (HCG) in late pregnancy. In multiple pregnancy the placenta is larger, and in molar pregnancy the uterus is filled with little but actively growing chorionic villi. After the third stage of labour is over, the condition begins to clear up as the cause of the hormonal imbalance is removed.

That the adrenal gland hypertrophies in all pregnancies has been known for generations, and pregnancy has been referred to as a physiological *Cushing's syndrome*. Corticosteroid production is more than doubled in pregnancy, and this will lead to hypertension. Why then does every pregnant woman not develop hypertension? The healthy placenta, it was stated, elaborated *monoamine oxidases* which counteracted the effects of the increased corticosteroids. In pre-eclampsia, however, a reduced placental blood flow caused reduced oxidase production as a result of which adrenal hypertrophy became clinically manifest.

That placental ischaemia is associated with pre-eclampsia is now generally accepted, but whether it is a cause or effect of the condition is debatable. The trophoblast may form a vasoconstrictor substance which unless counteracted causes vasospasm in the arterioles supplying the uterus. Studies on chorionic villi show that ischaemic changes may cause the release of thromboplastin which initiates *disseminated intravascular coagulation* (DIC) and deposition of fibrin (see page

160). This fibrinoid change in the villi which is much increased in severe pre-eclampsia may have an immunological basis.

The aetiology of one of the commonest and most important complications of pregnancy thus still remains obscure. In addition to altered humoral, hormonal and blood coagulation factors, nutritional defects may play a part in pre-eclampsia.

Clinical features of pre-eclampsia

The clinical manifestations of the conditions are shown diagrammatically in Figure 43. Accidental antepartum haemorrhage as a complication is discussed in Chapter 17, but further consideration of the clinical features, their significance and treatment is necessary.

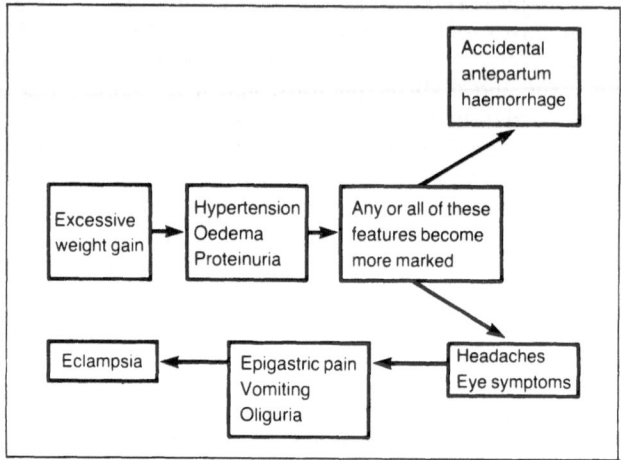

Figure 43   The clinical features of pre-eclamptic toxaemia

EXCESSIVE WEIGHT GAIN

In every pregnancy there is a tendency to retain sodium, and thus water, in the tissues, but this is more marked in pre-eclampsia where, in addition, spasm in the afferent glomerular arterioles leads to a reduction in renal blood flow and glomerular filtration.

Before excess water retention becomes clinically evident, it may be suggested by excessive weight gain, also referred to as *occult oedema*. Weight gain varies considerably in normal pregnancies and is generally slight in the first month. Thereafter, 2 kg in any 4 weeks should be the upper limit and, indeed, in the last month the normal patient often loses weight. If weight gain is excessive, the practitioner should look for finger oedema (are rings too tight?) and this is of significance especially when found early in the last trimester of pregnancy.

Patients who have gained too much weight should be advised to adopt a restful regime, take a high protein diet and restrict the intake of carbohydrates and salt (it is unnecessary, however, to restrict the latter drastically).

As far as rest is concerned, advice given should be such that the patient can accept and follow. Thus her social conditions, the number and ages of her children and whether or not they are at school, the availability of domestic help and support of relatives and friends, are important factors that will affect the amount of rest a patient is able to take.

Practical advice regarding shopping expeditions and housework given in terms such as 'do what you must and no more' and 'sit with your feet up whenever possible' is useful, and bedrest for an hour or two during the day is of considerable value. It is important to ensure that the patient does not miss her next prenatal check which should be earlier than that routinely given.

OEDEMA

Oedema affects legs, hands, face and abdominal wall (when, for example, the indent of a fetal stethoscope may still be visible seconds after use) and occasionally the vulva will suddenly become markedly oedematous. Rest is now vital. Diuretics generally should be avoided. Although sodium is retained in pregnancy, the increase in plasma volume is proportionally greater and this may lead to hyponatraemia; diuretics increase this tendency and do not in any way help the fetus. Indeed, the use of these drugs could lull patient and attendant into a sense of false security by masking an important symptom. If diuretics are used to eliminate severe oedema and thereby increase the comfort of the patient, it is essential to be even more watchful for other signs of pre-eclampsia. It is preferable to restrict the use of diuretics to patients under observation in hospital.

Hypertension, oedema and proteinuria are the three classical features of pre-eclampsia, and any one, or any combination of these manifestations, may indicate the presence of the condition.

HYPERTENSION

Hypertension as a sign of pre-eclampsia generally appears during the second half of pregnancy, so the practitioner will usually have several earlier recordings by which the patient's normal blood pressure range may be assessed.

It is impossible to make hard and fast rules concerning the level of blood pressure recordings in pre-eclampsia, but certain guiding principles can be given. The belief that there is no need for action if the recording does not exceed 140/90 is not without danger. These two figures are used arbitrarily as a basis for making a diagnosis of essential hypertension which may be made if two readings at or above this level are recorded in the first 20 weeks of pregnancy.

Essential hypertension

This is a disorder affecting the blood vessels and is associated with a generalized hypertonia or spasm of the arterioles. There may be a family history of hypertensive disorder. The condition in its benign much more common form should not be associated with evidence of renal insufficiency, and on the whole the prognosis in pregnancy for mother and baby is good. Tests for impairment of renal function have been discussed above (see page 64). The patient with essential hypertension is, however, more likely to develop a superimposed pre-eclampsia, as is the patient with a very labile blood pressure. Thus a restful regime throughout pregnancy is indicated and the patient should be seen more frequently than is normal and at least every 2 weeks in the early months. If there is any tendency for the hypertension to increase, hospitalization is advisable.

Blood pressure is best recorded with the patient seated. This obviates a false reading due to hypotension associated with compression of the inferior vena cava against the spinal column when the patient is supine, and which is not uncommon in the latter months of pregnancy.

NORMAL BLOOD PRESSURE AND PRE-ECLAMPSIA

It is impossible to give exact figures to represent the normal blood pressure in pregnancy as individual variation is considerable. The age of the patient is an influential factor and a lower recording for a teenager than for a patient approaching 40 would be anticipated. As a guide, a systolic recording of 100 to 135 and a diastolic pressure of 65 to 85 may be considered the normal range. There will, of course, be patients whose blood pressure is 90/60 or lower, and who are not subject to syncopal attacks or have any other problem, so each patient must be assessed individually. The blood pressure recording at the initial examination is one early recording, and it must be noted that there is a tendency for blood pressure to fall in the mid-trimester of pregnancy in many patients.

However, by the 20th week, or very shortly afterwards, there should be at least four recordings of blood pressure available to indicate the level for the individual. Any rise of this level should be regarded as significant, and if the rise is only slight the patient is advised to rest and a further check made within a few days. If blood pressure has not returned to its normal range by then very careful observation is essential.

Hospitalization should be considered when there is a rise in the normal diastolic blood pressure of about 15 points in a patient who had earlier been normotensive. A rise of less than this may indicate the need for institutional supervision in a patient with essential hypertension. The systolic recording, the actual level of blood pressure, other manifestations of disease and social conditions must all be taken into account.

PROTEINURIA

The causes of proteinuria in pregnancy were discussed in Chapter 6. As a manifestation of pre-eclampsia, proteinuria indicates the presence of considerable spasm in the afferent glomerular arterioles and is often associated with marked hypertension. The fetus is at risk and careful observation of mother and fetus in hospital is essential.

Manifestations of severe pre-eclampsia

HEADACHES

These are severe, throbbing and intractable. They may be frontal, on the crown of the head or occipital. The patient may be photophobic. If a simple analgesic such as soluble aspirin eases the headache, it is not due to pre-eclampsia.

VISUAL DISTURBANCES

These include flashing lights, blurring and diplopia as well as spots before the eyes. Patients who will have been advised to report certain symptoms immediately may seek advice about 'spots before the eyes' (this advice is included in the booklet given to all expectant mothers and mentioned on page 46. (Other symptoms patients are advised to report include headaches, fainting, swelling of feet, hand or face, abdominal pain and vaginal bleeding). Most people can become conscious of spots or 'shapes' which float across the field of vision, especially when looking at a bright background. These are normal and provided blood pressure and all else is normal, the patient can be reassured. If, however, she had become markedly hypertensive and complained of similar spots, the symptom must be investigated. The retina should be examined periodically in toxaemia although abnormal vascular changes are not found very often.

EPIGASTRIC PAIN

This pain found in severe pre-eclampsia is well localized, but the reason for it is unclear. It may be associated with cloudy swelling of the liver found in this condition.

VOMITING

Vomiting in pregnancy can be due to a variety of causes and may sometimes be iatrogenic, especially if morphine, for example, has been used.

OLIGURIA

This indicates impending renal failure and this may occur especially after eclamptic fits. Anuria would indicate the urgent necessity for the patient to be cared for by specialist staff in a renal unit.

Treatment of pre-eclampsia

The dietetic aspects of treatment have been mentioned in the discussion above, and the importance of rest cannot be overstressed. Bedrest will increase the blood supply to the uterus, except in some patients lying flat on their backs in whom may result hypotension. One very important aspect of hospitalization for pre-eclampsia is the careful observations made by the midwives and recorded on a chart, which should include:

(1)   Blood pressure, which is taken at least twice daily. Too frequent recordings may cause the patient some concern, but in severe cases monitoring is essential.
(2)   Quantitative estimations of proteinuria, if present.
(3)   The degree of oedema.
(4)   Any other manifestation.
(5)   Fluid intake and output. There is only an indirect relationship between fluid intake and fluid in the tissues, and it is unnecessary to restrict fluids drastically in an oedematous patient. More than a litre of fluid is lost daily through breath, skin and bowel. Thus intake for a day may be nearly 1 litre more than the previous 24 hours output and the patient is still losing fluid (that is, has a positive diuresis).

Fetal assessment

In addition to these observations and the general condition of the mother, a constant assessment of the fetus *in utero* is made. Fetal growth and maturity as measured by ultrasonography, tests for placental and fetal wellbeing, such as the 24-hour urinary oestriol estimation, and amnioscopy and amniocentesis (for example, for the lecithin–sphingomyelin ratio), are discussed below (Chapter 20).

Observations kept on both patient and fetus are the vital factors that will help the obstetrician to make the important decision regarding the optimum time to recommend termination of the pregnancy. If the pregnancy is in its last few weeks, the fetus is mature with head entering the pelvis and the cervix is 'ripe', the recommendation for labour to be induced need not be delayed. It is in cases where the pre-eclampsia is increasing in severity in spite of treatment in hospital and the fetus is markedly preterm that judgement is more difficult. It requires experience to judge whether a small, dysmature, preterm infant would be better delivered than left *in utero*. The tests mentioned above are most useful aids to clinical judgement (see Chapter 20).

Rest, careful observations, correct timing and mode of delivery and care of the neonate are the important features to help reduce perinatal mortality associated with pre-eclampsia. They are often more important than drug therapy, which includes:

(1) Sedatives
(2) Hypotensive reagents which may be indicated in essential hypertension, but also in pre-eclampsia
(3) Diuretics, the dangers and use of which have been discussed above.

Sedatives and hypotensive agents are discussed on page 142.

15

Eclampsia

Eclampsia is a condition associated with convulsions indistin-guishable from the fits of epilepsy. Proper prenatal care, the recogni-tion of the early warning signs and the correct management of pre-eclampsia should greatly reduce the incidence of this dangerous condi-tion. Eclampsia, however, may occur with dramatic suddenness in patients who, only a few days earlier, were normotensive with no obstetric complications. In about 50% of cases the first fit occurs before the onset of labour, but the initial convulsion may well be either intrapartum or postpartum. The risk of eclampsia occurring for the first time more than 48 hours after delivery is very slight.

Eclamptic fits
Eclamptic fits vary in intensity and may be transient phenomena akin to a minor form of petit mal. Major fits, however, result in loss of consciousness for hours, and in *status eclampticus* fit follows fit and the lives of both mother and baby are in jeopardy. The latter, fortun-ately, is extremely rare in the United Kingdom.

The convulsion itself may or may not be preceded by a prodromal phase during which the patient may cry out, twitch slightly or roll her eyes. Thereafter five phases can be distinguished:

(1) *The tonic stage*, characterized by rigidity and stillness. The muscles of the entire body go into spasm and the back arches. Spasm of the glottis occurs, respiration ceases and the patient rapidly becomes cyanosed.
(2) *The clonic stage* follows with its jactitations. In a minor fit the twitching may involve only the hands, eyes or mouth, but in a major episode it spreads rapidly to the entire body. Saliva fills the mouth and the convulsive movements of the jaw and tongue lather it into a froth which may be bloodstained if the patient bites her tongue.

(3) *Coma* ensues and is associated with deep sighing respiration or stertorous breathing. This stage passes into

(4) *Semicoma*, which is followed by

(5) *Natural sleep.*

Stages (3), (4) and (5) are all stages of insensibility. A patient cannot be roused from coma, but from semicoma she might give an animal response, and from sleep she should be able to respond normally. Since any stimulus whatsoever to a patient in these stages may well precipitate another fit, the division is purely academic. Each stage lasts longer than its predecessor and a clonic stage lasting over 60 seconds would indicate a major fit.

During an eclamptic convulsion a patient may die from asphyxia (by 'swallowing' her tongue), cerebral haemorrhage or acute heart failure. Later causes of death include renal and liver failure, hypostatic pneumonia and other intercurrent infections.

TREATMENT OF AN ECLAMPTIC FIT

All patients in hospital with severe pre-eclampsia require a trained member of staff in constant attendance day and night. They are nursed in a quiet room where all the equipment necessary for dealing with a fit should be immediately available. The patient must be protected from injury during a convulsion and the most important immediate duty of the attendant is to ensure a clear airway. A gag is inserted into the mouth at the onset of a convulsion and the tongue is kept forward if necessary with the aid of a tongue forceps. The gag may be a wooden wedge, a well-padded metal spatula or a Mason's gag, but its insertion may be difficult and trauma must be avoided. Oxygen is administered and frothy saliva removed by suction with the patient being nursed on her side.

Treatment of eclampsia

The basic aim of treatment is first to stop the fits and when this control is achieved to deliver the baby. Other measures include the reduction of hypertension, elimination of retained fluids and electrolytes, maintenance of adequate oxygenation of mother and fetus, and the prevention of infection. As a convulsion itself is associated with an abnormal discharge of impulses from the brain, stimuli should be prevented from arriving there by nursing the patient in a quiet, warm, partially darkened room, and the sensitivity of the brain diminished by sedation. Methods used vary considerably and newer drugs and regimes have now replaced the older ones. Each obstetrician tends to use the methods that his own experience has shown to be effective and the discussion that follows is not intended to provide a comprehensive list of drugs used today in the treatment of pre-eclampsia and eclampsia, but it includes mainly those that have been used by the author. Some older methods are also mentioned, as availability of drugs varies from area to area.

PARENTERAL THERAPY

When a patient has had an eclamptic fit, there is an urgent need for potent and effective parenteral therapy to stop further convulsions. Several treatment regimes of value are available today.

Diazepam (Valium) 10–20 mg intravenously

This is injected very slowly (taking at least 2 to 4 minutes) and the patient is observed closely as she rapidly becomes drowsy. This may sometimes be followed by an intravenous infusion containing 40 mg diazepam in 500 ml of 5% dextrose, the drip rate being controlled according to the needs of the patient; 10 mg intramuscularly every 4–6 hours is also very useful in severe cases.

Chlormethiazole edisylate (Heminevrin, 0.8% infusion)

Personal experience with this hypnotic and anticonvulsant drug has shown it to be very effective. The intravenous infusion is initially allowed to run in at 60 drops per minute and is slowed down immediately the patient appears drowsy. The drip rate is altered according to the patient's needs and may often fall below 10 drops per minute.

Paraldehyde 5–10 ml intramuscularly

This is an old, good and effective method of preventing recurrent fits. Paraldehyde has little toxicity and the patient is hardly likely to be bothered by its smell! The drug may be of particular value when administered by her doctor to a patient who has had a convulsion in her home and who is to be transferred to hospital. It must be noted, however, that an intramuscular injection of more than 5 ml (8 ml is the amount given to a pregnant woman of average stature) is painful and the pain itself may precipitate a fit. So it needs to be given slowly, possibly in divided doses.

Hydralazine hydrochloride (Apresoline)

Administered intravenously this agent lowers the blood pressure by causing peripheral vasodilatation and thereby improves renal, uterine and cerebral blood flow. An ampoule containing 20 mg of powder is reconstituted with 1 ml water and injected slowly. It may be further diluted in sodium chloride solution (but not dextrose) and given as an infusion. Tachycardia, headaches and nausea may follow its use. One 25 mg tablet three times a day is an average oral dose.

Frusemide (Lasix) 50 mg in 5 ml
Given intravenously and slowly this agent is used occasionally to promote diuresis.

OLDER TREATMENT REGIMES
Although these are not often used, they will be of interest to the student.

Morphine and chloral hydrate
The so-called *Stroganoff* regime using morphine hypodermically and chloral hydrate orally (or rectally) has probably saved countless thousands of lives all over the world. Adequate quantities of the two drugs were given to ensure that the patient did not have a further convulsion. Morphine depresses the respiratory centre, so should not be repeated if the patient's respiratory rate falls below 17 bpm. In its day the regime was very good, but morphine is not an effective anticonvulsant and the nausea or vomiting that some patients experience as its effect diminishes may also precipitate a fit.

Hypertonic solutions of magnesium sulphate
These were administered intramuscularly or intravenously. The drug was first used when in an endeavour to eliminate the 'toxin' concentrated solutions of the compound (Epsom Salts) were placed in the stomach to act as a purgative. Results were good but unrelated to purgation! Magnesium acts on the neuromuscular junction, the hypertonic solution removes fluids from the tissues and promotes diuresis and, by a combination of these features the blood pressure may be lowered. One regime thus employed was 4 ml of 50% magnesium sulphate given intramuscularly every 6 hours for four doses. This, used in combination with other sedatives (see below), was found to be most effective therapy, especially during labour.

OTHER HYPOTENSIVE DRUGS
Other hypotensive drugs used include methyldopa (Aldomet) and propranolol (Inderal), a beta-adrenergic receptor blocking drug. Diazoxide, clonidine and other ganglion blockers are also used. Protoveratrine, rauwolfia extracts and veratrum viride have all been used in the past, and bromethol (Avertin) rectally is still used by many with good effect.

Sedation in pre-eclampsia and eclampsia
Other forms of sedation used in pre-eclampsia and eclampsia may include the following.

BARBITURATES
Patients' reactions to barbiturates vary from individual to individual and it is preferable to avoid this group of drugs. Amylobarbitone (Amytal) as a sedative in small doses, such as 30–50 mg 8-hourly or 100–200 mg at night may be of value in pre-eclampsia.

STRONGER SEDATIVES
Those used in hospital in severe pre-eclampsia include 'cocktails' for intramuscular injection every 6–8 hours. They contain 25–50 mg of promethazine hydrochloride (Phenergan), promazine hydrochloride (Sparine) and possibly chlorpromazine hydrochloride (Largactil). When labour ensues, pethidine or pethidine with levallorphan (Pethilorfan) may be substituted for promethazine.

Management during labour
When eclamptic fits are under control, the pregnancy is terminated usually by surgical induction of labour, although caesarean section is considered if conditions for induction and vaginal delivery are unfavourable. Epidural analgesia may be administered at this stage and carefully monitored during the ensuing labour. During treatment the patient's fluid and electrolyte balance are watched, and although intravenous feeding is the rule, oral fluids are sometimes given in less severe cases. A full bladder can precipitate a convulsion and it is often necessary to insert a Foley catheter and institute continuous bladder drainage. Bowels are ignored.

During labour sedation is increased as necessary, and delivery is usually assisted as the patient must not be allowed to push in the second stage, although spontaneous delivery occasionally occurs quite easily. The third stage is managed normally, and the patient must be kept well sedated for at least 48 hours after delivery.

16

Vomiting in pregnancy and hyperemesis gravidarum

As has been stated above (page 42) nausea can affect approximately 50% of women at some stage of a pregnancy. So-called 'morning sickness', seen generally between the 6th and 16th weeks, occurs at varying times during the day and also varies in severity. In its mildest form the condition may be manifest as a transient bout of nausea on rising from bed, the patient remaining fit for the rest of the 24 hours, or nausea may occur in the evening. As the severity of the condition increases the frequency of the bouts of nausea increases and there is vomiting. A patient may vomit once during the day or after taking solid foods, and in the most severe forms of the condition she is unable to retain even small amounts of fluid. When vomiting of pregnancy affects physical health the condition is called *hyperemesis gravidarum.*

The aetiology is not established and although removing sufferers to hospital away from the family environment is sometimes effective, the condition is not wholly psychological in origin. Adaptation to the physical, humoral and hormonal changes due to pregnancy plays its part, and vomiting centres in the brain have been described. In the most severe form the condition can be dangerous but fortunately this is rare. Women can be affected in varying degrees or not at all in successive pregnancies whether planned or unplanned.

The most important advice to give to the patient with mild 'morning sickness' is to avoid situations of stress, to rise slowly and gently from bed and to have frequent light 'snacks' of carbohydrate rather than fatty foods. If sickness occurs in the morning, the patient is advised to have tea (or any other beverage she prefers), preferably sweetened to taste, with a dry biscuit, before rising. The patient who is awakened suddenly by an alarm clock and hurriedly jumps out of bed is much more likely to vomit.

Drug therapy is best avoided in the first 4 months of pregnancy whenever possible. Barbiturates used extensively in the past with effect should be withheld. Antihistamines such as promethazine 25 mg

145

at night or meclozine 25–50 mg (with or without pyridoxine) have helped many patients, but the principle of prescribing drugs in early pregnancy *only when essential* should be observed at all times. At the time of writing a drug used widely in the United Kingdom and the United States is the subject of litigation.

When vomiting is troublesome other conditions must be considered and eliminated as a causative factor. Conditions in which vomiting is a symptom are legion, but most will have other manifestations to alert the practitioner to the fact that something other than an intrauterine pregnancy is responsible. Any pyrexial condition, acute gastroenteritis or specific fever may be associated, or the clinical picture may be that of an acute addomen – caused by perhaps acute appendicitis, cholecystitis, pancreatitis or ectopic pregnancy. Some conditions such as duodenal ulcer or hiatus hernia may be aggravated by pregnancy and cause symptoms, while others related to the pregnant state include:

(1)   Torsion in an ovarian cyst.
(2)   Pyelonephritis.
(3)   Degeneration in a fibroid (usually in later pregnancy).
(4)   Abruptio placentae.
(5)   Hepatic disorders (acute fatty liver of pregnancy or acute yellow atrophy, and a condition called *obstetric hepatosis* are rare complications that occur in the last trimester).
(6)   Severe pre-eclampsia, which although usually seen late in pregnancy occurs earlier when associated with multiple pregnancy, acute hydramnios or hydatidiform mole.

Most of these conditions are discussed elsewhere in this book (Chapters 6 and 14). The possibility that vomiting may be associated with or aggravated by drugs, alcohol, nasal and chest infections in which secretion may be swallowed should also be considered.

When vomiting in pregnancy is not controlled by measures discussed above, and the patient shows evidence of dehydration and ketosis, hospitalization becomes necessary. Some women may improve immediately, as already stated, and staff should ensure that visitors do not show anxiety when with the patient (a vomit bowl, although available, is better kept out of sight!)

Dehydration may be readily apparent and the patient's tongue is dry and furred. Urine passed is concentrated and in addition to ketone bodies may contain protein and bile.

Sedation may need to be increased. In addition to those already mentioned, drugs such as diazepam (5 mg intramuscularly), prochlorperazine (12.5 mg intramuscularly and/or Stemetil rectal suppositories), and promazine (intramuscularly or intravenously – for example, 25–50 mg in glucose–saline solution) may be used. A record of fluid intake and output is kept, and investigations should include serum electrolytes and liver function tests. Intravenous drip feeding with 10% glucose–saline (3 litres at least in 24 hours) is initiated. Ice may be sucked to keep the buccal mucosa moist.

When vomiting is controlled oral feeding is reintroduced slowly, starting initially with small quantities of fluid. Light meals, largely of carbohydrates in the first place, may be given, but the patient's own preferences should be heeded when possible.

Hyperemesis gravidarum is an excessively rare indication for termination of pregnancy.

17

Haemorrhages of pregnancy

Haemorrhages from the genital tract occur in both early and late pregnancy. In the United Kingdom the division between the two takes place at the 28th week, the time at which, according to statute, the fetus becomes viable or capable of a separate existence. With modern methods of fetal resuscitation and intensive neonatal care, many babies born before the 28th week can and do survive. The timing of viability by law has assumed considerable importance in view of the vast increase in numbers of therapeutic terminations of pregnancy performed following the Abortion Act of 1967. Other countries, and some states in the United States, adopted a World Health Organization recommendation that viability commenced at 20 weeks, and some authorities prefer fetal weight to be the criterion. There must be very few who do not consider, on medical grounds, that the statutory 28 weeks in the United Kingdom should be reduced. Much debate recently in Parliament on suggested amendments to the law concerning abortion has currently not resulted in any alteration, although there is every prospect that the legal definition of viability will be changed in the not-too-distant future. Opinion, medical and parliamentary, appears to differ between 20 and 24 weeks.

Abortion or miscarriage (the words are synonymous) and other causes of bleeding in the first 28 weeks of pregnancy are topics which may be considered more suitable for a gynaecology rather than obstetrics textbook. However, the two disciplines are closely interwoven, and certainly knowledge of the causes of bleeding throughout pregnancy from beginning to end is necessary for all participating in maternal care.

Haemorrhage in early pregnancy
There are five main causes of bleeding from the genital tract in early pregnancy.

(1) *Decidual bleeding* (Figure 44). This is a shedding of the decidua vera (page 32) and may be the cause of slight blood loss at the time of expected menstruation up to the 3rd month of pregnancy. The diagnosis is purely of academic interest as it should be made only in retrospect, since at the time of its occurrence the loss must be regarded as a threat to abort. Decidual bleeding mistaken for a normal period may cause errors in estimating the date of delivery.

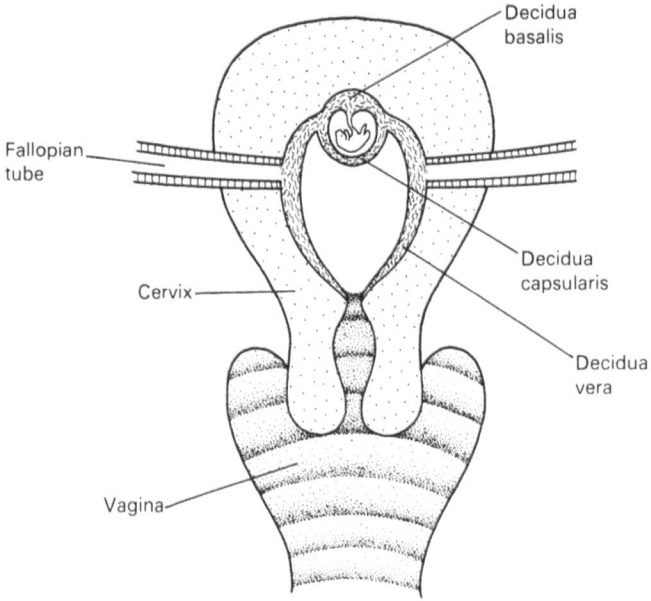

Figure 44   Decidual bleeding. The decidua vera may shed without disturbing the pregnancy

(2) *Abortion in all its types.*
(3) *Ectopic pregnancy.*
(4) *Hydatidiform mole.*
(5) *Extrauterine bleeding,* such as may occur from cervical polypi or erosions, varicose veins, or (rarely) in association with carcinoma of the cervix. Severe vaginitis may cause 'spotting' of blood. This type of bleeding may be excluded by examination with a vaginal speculum.

ABORTION
Abortion may be defined as an attempt to expel, or the active expulsion of the uterine contents before the 28th week of pregnancy. (The

timing of 28 weeks is subject to the provisos on viability as discussed above, and the definition does not necessarily include cases of missed abortion). The incidence of spontaneous abortion is difficult to determine. Many women may have had an early abortion without knowing it and others claim that a pregnancy existed when in fact menstruation had been delayed for some other reason. However, approximately 20% of all pregnancies terminate by spontaneous abortion. The more important causes of abortion with essentials of management are discussed below.

Fetal abnormalities
This category includes the abnormal zygote (the term 'abnormal ovum' is a misnomer as the fault may lie in the spermatazoon), and genetic or chromosomal defects. The aetiological factors responsible for the abnormality are often obscure. The age of the ovum when fertilized, maternal age, drugs and virus infections, may be considered. Hydatidiform mole changes are often present in the chorionic tissue. There may be no fetus or a whitish speck in the fetal sac may represent the 'blighted ovum'.

The belief that abortion may be the means by which nature eliminates the abnormal leads some authorities to recommend that no measures be taken when abortion threatens. Personal experience, however, is that if a threatened abortion is associated with an abnormal fetus the pregnancy will terminate anyway in spite of complete bedrest, which should be recommended in all cases.

Uterine abnormalities
The following may be causes.

(1)   *Fibroids* which may distort the uterine cavity.
(2)   Developmental abnormalities such as the *bicornuate uterus* (see page 121).
(3)   *Retrodisplacement of the uterus* could be a factor but in fact rarely plays a part. Certainly any attempt to manipulate a gravid uterus forward is more likely to disturb the pregnancy than the original retrodisplacement. As stated in Chapter 4 the best advice to patients is to avoid excessive activity, to abstain from coitus when menstruation would normally be expected, and occasionally to adopt the prone attitude without causing discomfort to themselves. These simple precautions are taken until the 14th or 15th week by which time the uterus is an abdominal organ and cannot displace backwards, and the placenta is well localized.

Acute retention of urine, due to impaction or incarceration of the retroverted gravid uterus at approximately 12 weeks gestation, is uncommon and easily dealt with by slow decompression of the bladder by catheterization.

(4) *Severe cervical tears and the so-called 'incompetent os'*. Repair (or *trachelorrhaphy*) may sometimes be indicated where old cervical lacerations are considered to be a factor in abortion. The incompetent internal os is a cause of abortion after the 12th week of pregnancy when the fetal sac fills the uterine cavity and herniates into the cervical canal initiating labour. Insertion of a suture with, say, nylon tape at the level of the internal os (*Shirodkar suture*) takes a few minutes and is most effective in selected cases.

Endocrine and vitamin deficiencies

The corpus luteum is essential to the maintenance of early pregnancy in nearly all animals. Emergency removal of the ovary containing this body in women in the first trimester of pregnancy, however, does not always lead to abortion. Progesterone deficiency was considered to be a likely contributory cause of unsuccessful pregnancy and doses of the hormone were administered. Attempts to rationalize this treatment by estimating the excretion product in urine (*pregnanediol*) were made. It was also thought that progesterone inhibited the motility of uterine muscle. However, the use of all hormones in pregnancy is contraindicated.

Deficiency of folic acid and other substances such as vitamin B_{12} which are necessary for the synthesis of nucleic acids may be a factor in abortion.

Trauma

This may be directly or indirectly applied. Direct trauma by injury to the uterus via the abdominal wall must be a very rare cause of abortion. Furthermore, a properly implanted ovum should be proof against strenuous muscular effort applied as a possible form of indirect trauma. Instrumentation via the vagina and cervical canal is the most common traumatic cause of abortion.

Maternal illnesses and diseases

(1) *Acute.* Any pyrexial condition such as influenza, pyelitis and the specific fevers may be responsible for abortion.

(2) *Chronic* conditions which may affect the chorionic tissue include diabetes mellitus, syphilis, chronic nephritis and some severe chronic anaemias (for example, those associated with ankylostomiasis seen in the tropics).

Induced abortion

This may be brought about by the use of drugs or instrumentation and may be therapeutic or criminal.

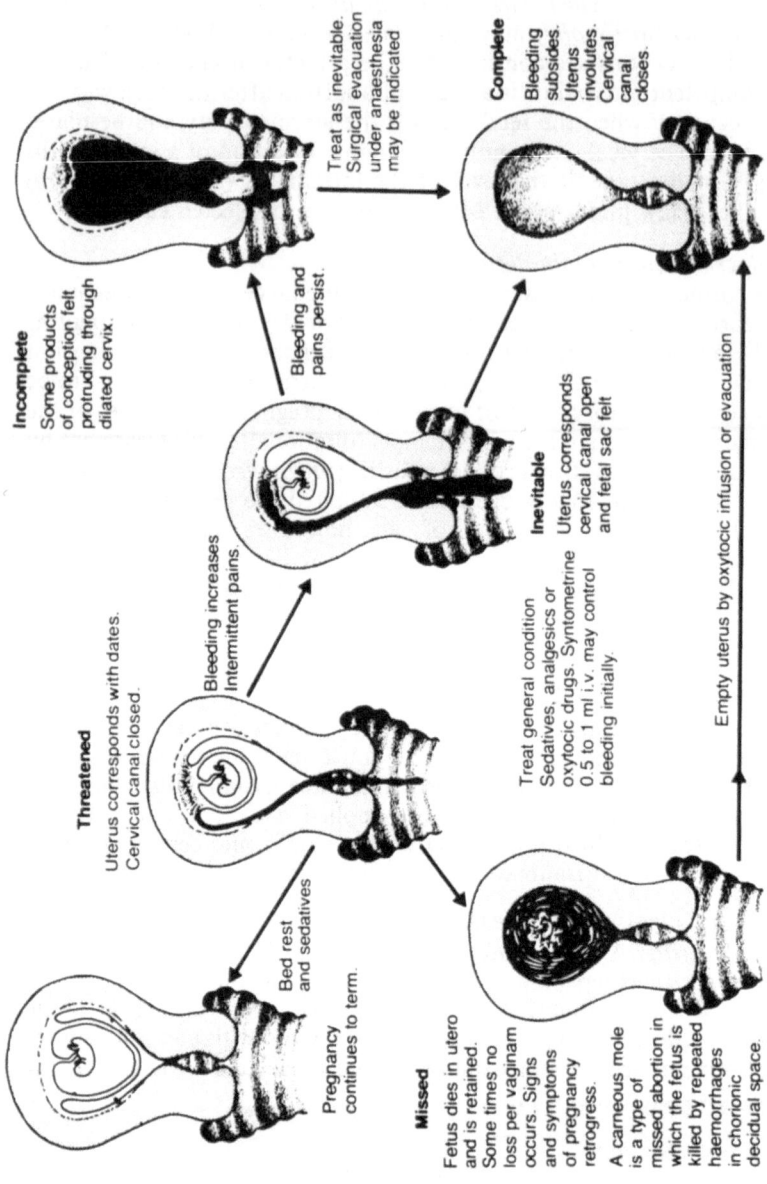

Threatened
Uterus corresponds with dates. Cervical canal closed.

Pregnancy continues to term.

Bed rest and sedatives

Incomplete
Some products of conception felt protruding through dilated cervix.

Bleeding increases Intermittent pains.

Bleeding and pains persist.

Treat as inevitable. Surgical evacuation under anaesthesia may be indicated

Complete
Bleeding subsides. Uterus involutes. Cervical canal closes.

Inevitable
Uterus corresponds cervical canal open and fetal sac felt

Treat general condition Sedatives, analgesics or oxytocic drugs. Syntometrine 0.5 to 1 ml i.v. may control bleeding initially.

Empty uterus by oxytocic infusion or evacuation

Missed
Fetus dies in utero and is retained. Some times no loss per vaginam occurs. Signs and symptoms of pregnancy retrogress.

A carneous mole is a type of missed abortion in which the fetus is killed by repeated haemorrhages in chorionic decidual space.

Figure 45   The clinical features and types of abortion

The clinical types of abortion and indications as to management are shown in Figure 45. In most cases of abortion the patient has signs and symptoms of early pregnancy, and then vaginal bleeding occurs before pain. In the first 12 weeks, when the fetal sac is surrounded by active chorionic villi, vaginal bleeding always occurs as an early symptom. After the 12th week, the clinical features of abortion may be akin to those of normal labour, that is, the process may begin with 'pains' or by rupture of the membranes with a loss of liquor prior to a show of bloodstained mucus.

ECTOPIC PREGNANCY

An ectopic pregnancy (from the Greek word for 'out of place') is one which develops elsewhere than in the decidua of the uterine cavity. Most such pregnancies embed in the fallopian tubes and, much less commonly, in the ovary, uterine cornua or cervix. A primary abdominal pregnancy in which a spermatozoon fertilizes an ovum and the zygote develops in the abdominal cavity is a very rare occurrence; so tubal ectopic pregnancy only is considered here. The aetiology of the condition is generally obscure although previous salpingitis may be a factor. Experience has also shown an increase in the incidence of tubal pregnancy when an intrauterine contraceptive device (IUD) is in place, and there is approximately a 10% increased risk of a second tubal pregnancy in a patient who has had one previously.

The possibility of ectopic pregnancy must be considered in every woman with abdominal pain who may be pregnant, and this must include very young people too. Clinically, manifestations of early pregnancy (especially delay in expected menstruation) are followed by recurrent bouts of abdominal pain often associated with nausea and faintness. Shoulder pain may be experienced if blood leaks upwards to the diaphragm when the patient is recumbent. Vaginal bleeding comes after the pain – a reversal of the sequence found in most cases of abortion.

The sequence of events is explained as follows and it will be readily appreciated if the physiology of the menstrual cycle and early development described in Chapter 2 are understood.

The trophoblast (early chorionic villi) attaches itself to the thin mucosa lining the tube. These attachments are insecure, and each time some of the villi detach themselves, bleeding occurs in the tube. The blood leaks from the abdominal ostium of the tube and may collect in the pouch of Douglas, causing pain. Eventually, when sufficient villi separate for the fetus to die, and there is no longer a continuing pregnancy, the corpus luteum atrophies. The withdrawal of the ovarian hormones results in a shedding of the thickened secretory decidua, in other words there is vaginal bleeding. If the decidua is shed *en masse*, the product passed is the '*decidual cast*', but more commonly it is shed in fragments.

Histologically the decidua will show marked secretory changes, but there will, of course, be no evidence of trophoblastic tissue.

Blood in the pelvis leads to acute tenderness, and abdominal examination may show the tenderness and guarding to be more marked in one or other of the iliac fossae. Bimanually, the practitioner may be able to feel a slightly bulky uterus and appreciate a very tender tubal swelling, but often the tenderness is so marked that tubal palpation is impossible. The patient will also experience severe pain when the cervix is gently rocked to and fro. A gentle examination is essential and the risk of rupturing the tube is present and increased if the gynaecologist performs the examination under anaesthesia. Rupture of the ectopic pregnancy may result in profuse internal haemorrhage and will give rise to severe pain, marked abdominal tenderness and shock. Blood pressure falls with the shock, but quite often the pulse rate does not rise as might be expected. Experience has shown many women with litres of blood in the peritoneal cavity whose pulse rate has remained steady at, or below, 70 bpm. Spontaneous rupture of the tube may occur at an early stage if the fertilized ovum is implanted in the narrow tubal isthmus.

Many ectopic pregnancies are not diagnosed and may not require surgery. A woman may think a period has been delayed and then experience a variation in menstruation associated with pain which she considers to be severe dysmenorrhoea. In fact, she may have a tubal pregnancy which has died and is retained in the tube. Such a *tubal mole* may be absorbed.

Other possible outcomes of tubal pregnancy include *tubal abortion* which is said to have occurred when the fertilized ovum is discharged into the peritoneal cavity. The abortion may be complete or incomplete. Blood leaking from the fimbriated end of the tube may form a clotted mass in the pouch of Douglas or a *peritubal haematocoele*.

The fetus may survive if the chorionic villi erode slowly through the tube and attach to the omentum or gut. Such a *secondary abdominal pregnancy* may be intraperitoneal or intraligamentary if erosion takes place through the inferior aspect of the tube and between the layers of the broad ligament. A few babies have been known to survive after laparotomy but more often the fetus dies. On extremely rare occasions a fetus undergoes mummification (*adipocere* formation) or, as records show, becomes infected and forms abscesses and sinuses through which bones discharge. Medical museums contain *lithopaedions* — compact masses of bone which are the end result of calcification of abdominal pregnancy.

Aids to diagnosis
These include:

(1) Pregnancy test, which if positive indicates only the presence of living chorionic tissue in the body and no more.
(2) Laparoscopy.
(3) Culdocentesis, achieved by thrusting a needle with a syringe through the posterior fornix to ascertain whether blood is present in the pouch of Douglas.
(4) Examination under anaesthesia which must be performed with care to avoid rupturing the tube.
(5) Dilatation and curettage, which may be of some value.

However, taking an accurate history is most important in diagnosis, as a negative examination does not exclude the possibility of an ectopic pregnancy. The patient should be questioned regarding recent coitus, as in the presence of an active ectopic this would have been extremely painful if not impossible.

Treatment
With exception of an absorbing tubal mole, an ectopic pregnancy is removed at the earliest opportunity. In the general treatment of a shocked patient, rest, warmth, reassurance, and drug therapy with morphine, Omnopon (papaveretum) or pethidine are valuable. Above all, however, the shocked patient with tubal rupture will require urgent transfusion. At operation autotransfusion using filtered blood from the abdominal cavity of the patient may be a lifesaving measure if matched blood is not immediately available.

HYDATIDIFORM MOLE
Hydatidiform mole is essentially a trophoblastic neoplasm in which the fetus is blighted and the chorionic villi continue to multiply and undergo cystic change. The centre of the villus degenerates and fluid collects so that the villus begins to resemble a grape. Indeed, the condition is sometimes not diagnosed until the patient passes obviously molar tissue in the form of 'grapes' with a vaginal bleed.

Clinical features
The following features establish the diagnosis.

(1) Signs and symptoms of early pregnancy are followed by a vaginal bleed in which molar tissue is often found. Haemorrhage can be profuse and bright red in colour.

(2)   Hyperemesis gravidarum is more frequently seen than in a normal pregnancy.

(3)   Pre-eclampsia may occur. This is seen in the first half of pregnancy unlike other pregnancies in which pre-eclampsia tends to be a complication of the last trimester.

(4)   The uterus may be larger than dates suggest and have a 'doughy' feel. (The word 'doughy' used for decades by most textbooks to describe the feel of the uterus containing a mole remains apt). In 50% of cases, however, the uterus is not larger than anticipated and may correspond in size or even be smaller than suggested by menstrual history. It should be noted that there are varying grades of activity of hydatidiform mole, from an actively proliferating type to one in which degenerative changes predominate. The features being discussed are those associated with a typically active mole.

(5)   Ultrasonic echogram. At an early stage in the first trimester ultrasound scan produces a characteristic speckled appearance due to the echoes from the vesicles. The absence of a fetus is also to be noted.

(6)   Considerable quantities of chorionic gonadotrophin (HCG) are produced by the proliferating chorionic villi and the finding of excessive amounts in urine or in serum is an important means of establishing the diagnosis. Tests such as routine pregnancy tests in urine diluted to at least 1 in 100 have been replaced by radio-immune assays to estimate HCG quantitatively. The excessive quantity of this hormone may also stimulate the ovaries in which theca-lutein cysts develop. The cysts may become larger than a fetal head at term but retrogress after all mole tissue has been eliminated. High quantities of HCG are also found in normal twin pregnancies, and the possibility that molar changes can occur in only one conceptus may make the result of this test alone inconclusive.

Risks

The dangers of hydatidiform mole are:

(1)   Haemorrhage which can be profuse and cause profound shock.

(2)   Infection. An increased risk to all patients when anaemic and in whom operative procedures and repeated vaginal examinations are necessary.

(3)   Perforation of the wall of the uterus can occur as the mole may penetrate the myometrium. Benign moles can have invasive properties and metastasize in the lungs. These pulmonary deposits disappear when the molar condition is eliminated.

(4) Malignant change. The reported incidence of hydatidiform mole becoming the very malignant chorioncarcinoma varies from 2% to 10%.

The comparison between the development of the trophoblast and a malignant process has been made earlier (page 33) and the importance of the placenta as a structure for research into the processes of autoimmunology has been mentioned. That the condition is due to a breakdown of maternal—fetal immunological relationships is widely believed, and the fact that many women have had molar pregnancies with one husband and not with a second has led some researchers to stress the responsibility of paternal genes. In Europe and America the incidence of hydatidiform mole is about 1 in 2000 pregnancies, but the figure may be increased four to ten times in some Asian countries. Older primigravidae are more prone to develop the condition.

Treatment
Removal of all mole tissue is essential, yet it must be remembered that the uterine wall may be weakened and eroded so the danger of perforation at curettage is increased. The tendency when labour begins is for the uterus to empty itself, so initially medical means to achieve this are advisable. Oxytocic infusion is used and the strength of the solution may be increased regularly until uterine contractions are initiated. An infusion of prostaglandin which is a more potent agent than oxytocin is preferable. Blood transfusion, too, may be indicated to improve the patient's general condition.

Within 3 to 7 days of the expulsion of the mole, curettage is performed using a suction or large blunt curette. If any mole tissue is still present a second dilatation and curettage should be undertaken 7 to 10 days later. With the use of prostaglandin, abdominal hysterotomy is rarely necessary although abdominal hysterectomy is sometimes recommended.

Regular follow-up for a period of at least a year is conducted to ensure that the elimination of chorionic tissue is complete. Estimations of HCG by radioimmune assays made at weekly intervals should show a falling level to normality within 6 weeks. Thereafter monthly investigations may be enough. During the period of follow-up the patient must avoid a further pregnancy.

Chorioncarcinoma is best treated in specialized centres where available, and chemotherapy cures most cases. A generation ago the malignancy once established was usually fatal, and treatment by radical surgery and/or radiotherapy was of no use. Today folic acid antagonists such as methotrexate and other chemotherapeutic agents are used.

Haemorrhage in late pregnancy

The definitions that follow use the 28th week of pregnancy as the time factor for viability, but the remarks made in the opening paragraph of this chapter apply again. The classification used is considered the best but further comments on terminology are made.

Bleeding in late pregnancy may be due to any of the following four causes.

(1) *Accidental antepartum haemorrhage (Accidental APH)*. This may be defined as bleeding from the genital tract, after the 28th week of pregnancy and before the birth of the baby, from a placenta which is normally situated (that is, in the upper segment of the uterus). Excluded from this is the 'show' which generally heralds the onset of labour.

(2) *Unavoidable APH*. This is bleeding after the 28th week of pregnancy and before the birth of the baby from a placenta which is partly or wholly in the lower segment (placenta praevia).

(3) *APH of unestablished aetiology* which is either (1) or (2) above, when the exact situation of the placenta is not known. With modern facilities for placental localization in the United Kingdom today, this category is used less commonly.

(4) *Extrauterine bleeding*, the causes of which have already been mentioned (page 149).

ACCIDENTAL APH OR ABRUPTIO PLACENTAE

The normally implanted placenta should be secure against minor trauma which may be applied directly (such as by a fall or blow), or indirectly (such as by muscular effort). External cephalic version may be responsible for a small number of cases of placental separation, but this is unlikely if performed by an experienced and gentle practitioner. Occasionally haemorrhage may follow the rapid and sudden release of a copious quantity of liquor by rupture of the membranes in cases of hydramnios.

APH is initiated by a bleed in the decidua when a wall of a venous sinus in the placental area ruptures. The bleeding spreads immediately to the chorionic-decidual space causing placental separation. The blood shed may pass down in this space so that the entire loss becomes visible at the introitus. This is the *revealed* type of accidental APH. In some cases, however, the blood remains *in utero* distending the organ and passes between the muscle fibres so that the myometrium becomes disorganized. In severe cases the blood reaches the outer surface of the uterus and will detach areas of the peritoneum from its underlying muscle. This constitutes a *concealed* accidental APH, even though a small amount of blood often passes downwards in the chorionic-decidual space to show itself at the introitus. The swollen haemorrhagic uterus was first described by Couvelaire as uterine apoplexy (*apopléxie utéroplacentaire*).

The clinical features of the revealed and concealed forms of haemorrhage are quite different, but a third type occurs which combines features of the two. This is the *mixed* accidental APH in which much of the blood is revealed, but some is retained, and a localized area of the myometrium in the upper segment is disorganized by haematomata between the muscle fibres. This type is now more common in the United Kingdom than the severe classical type of concealed haemorrhage which kills the fetus and endangers the mother's life, and which was a complication of pregnancy seen more often in the tired, anaemic grandmultipara who had had little or no prenatal care.

Alternative classification of accidental APH
Some authorities suggest that the terms 'revealed', 'mixed' and 'concealed' for accidental APH be replaced by 'mild', 'moderate' and 'severe', depending upon features such as presence or absence of shock, blood pressure, area of uterine tenderness, amount of blood lost and the degree of placental separation. Some of these features cannot be measured with accuracy but there is merit in this classification and Table 1 gives many of the clinical features of the three types of accidental haemorrhage.

Table 1 Comparison of the clinical picture in the various grades of accidental haemorrhage (from Llewellyn-Jones (1977), with permission)*

	Mild	*Moderate*	*Severe*
Pulse	No change	Raised	Raised
Blood pressure	No change	Lowered	Lowered
Shock	None	Often	Always
Oliguria	Rare	Occasionally	Common
Hypofibrinogenaemia	Rare	Occasionally	Common
Uterus	Normal	Tender	Tender and tense
Fetus	Alive	Usually dead	Dead
Blood loss (in pints)	Less than 1	1 to 3	3 to 6

Other classifications have been recommended, and the term 'accidental' (now over 200 years old) has been dropped by some because it suggests a relationship to trauma. Most nurses and doctors in the United Kingdom use the terms 'revealed', 'concealed' and 'mixed' to describe the three types of accidental APH. There seems to be no good reason for altering the old terminology.

*Llewellyn-Jones, D. (1977). *Fundamentals of Obstetrics and Gynaecology, Vol. 1, 2nd edition.* (London: Faber and Faber).

Incidence

Accidental bleeding occurs in 1—2% of all pregnancies and is often associated with pre-eclampsia. The incidence of the latter as a complication of pregnancy increases with the severity of the bleed and is found in most cases of concealed haemorrhage.

Signs and symptoms

Revealed (mild) haemorrhage. The signs and symptoms of the revealed (mild) type of haemorrhage are those connected with blood loss together with those of pre-eclampsia, if present. In addition, backache or mild abdominal discomfort precedes the loss, but palpation reveals no abdominal tenderness. If the presenting part of the fetus is engaged (often the pregnancy has not advanced far enough for this to be so), the presence of placenta praevia may be discounted.

A typical case in the United Kingdom may present as a woman in the last trimester of pregnancy awakening in the morning with lower abdominal discomfort and losing blood vaginally while emptying her bladder. In reply to direct questioning the patient admits to backache the previous day and oedema of hands and feet over the past few days. Blood pressure may be elevated (or reduced if the revealed loss is heavy) and proteinuria may or may not be present.

A severe concealed haemorrhage. This manifests itself with shock and pain. The onset is sudden and the condition is often associated with severe toxaemia, so that a patient may have systolic blood pressure of around 200 at one moment which becomes difficult to record after the catastrophe. Proteinuria is common, and the shocked patient may vomit and/or have a rigor. The uterus becomes tense, woody hard, extremely tender and may become larger in minutes as blood collects within it. The fetus cannot be palpated and no heart sounds are present. The clinical picture presented may be one of an 'acute abdomen' and suggest a ruptured uterus. Amniotic fluid embolism associated with placental abruption in labour is reported and this may increase the shock. The degree of shock present is often more than might be anticipated by the estimated blood loss, and comparisons in the past have been made to the 'crush syndrome' which is also associated with much disorganization of muscle tissue.

Disseminated intravascular coagulation (DIC). Blood coagulation defects can arise in many obstetric complications and especially in association with severe concealed APH. Blood clotting essentially is is due to the conversion of the blood protein *fibrinogen* into threads of *fibrin*, a change brought about by the enzyme *thrombin*. The latter is formed from blood *prothrombin* when injured tissues and blood platelets liberate *thrombokinase* or *thromboplastin* in the presence of calcium. Many other factors are involved and normally blood clotting and anticlotting mechanisms are in balance. Following a concealed APH, extensive clotting retroplacentally and in the myometrium depletes fibrinogen in the blood and thromboplastin-like substances may be released and initiate a generalized coagulopathy known as disseminated intravascular coagulation (DIC). This disturbance is most complex but, in essence, it may be said that the formation and deposition of fibrin activates the normally protective fibrinolytic system. Fibrinolysis results in the release of *fibrin degradation products (FDPs)* which prevent platelet aggregation and tend to inhibit further clotting. Resultant hypofibrinogenaemia and a degree of thrombocytopenia lead to a vicious circle which presents as an increased tendency to haemorrhage.

Hypofibrinogenaemia may also occur in association with amniotic fluid embolus, retention of a dead fetus in utero, severe pre-eclampsia, hydatidiform mole and endotoxic shock seen in infections with Gram-negative organisms in septic abortions.

The mixed (moderate) accidental APH. Not unexpectedly this presents a clinical picture with some of the features of both the other grades. Although a moderate amount of blood passes downwards in the chorionic-decidual space to 'reveal' itself, some remains in utero and extravasation occurs into the muscle over a localized area. There is a degree of shock, and marked tenderness over the affected area of myometrium in the upper segment. The fetus may be felt and heart sounds may be audible. Pre-eclampsia is associated with up to 50% of cases of this type.

Treatment of antepartum haemorrhage
Every case of APH requires hospitalization for adequate management and observation. Bedrest for several days with no fresh bleeding is essential, even for cases where haemorrhage may appear to have been minimal. Crossmatched blood should be available at all times.

Mild revealed bleeding. After 48 hours rest, with sedation as required, the cervix and vagina are visualized with the aid of a speculum and extrauterine causes for the blood loss may thus be excluded. If the pregnancy has not progressed to the last month, the bleeding has settled, manifestations of pre-eclampsia are absent and there is no doubt that the placenta is situated in the upper segment, the patient may return home for continued rest. However, further prenatal examinations should be frequent and monitoring of placental efficiency is indicated.

If the pregnancy is in the last month, the fetal head is entering the pelvis or engaged and the cervix is 'ripe', it is preferable to perform induction of labour by artificial rupture of the membranes. This procedure usually stops further bleeding immediately and should be combined with oxytocic infusion.

Concealed haemorrhage. Prompt and adequate therapy to overcome hypovolaemic, haemorrhagic shock is essential. Transfusion with fresh whole blood should be liberal and fluid balance observed carefully as ischaemic renal damage may lead to renal failure. Central venous pressure (CVP) monitoring (in late pregnancy this should be about 10 cm water) is advisable to ensure adequate and correct fluid replacement. Sedation with, say, morphine is helpful. Early rupture of the forewaters and oxytocic infusion are indicated.

Infusion of fibrinogen will increase the deposition of fibrin, and fibrinolysis will lead to increased plasma levels of fibrin degradation products and should thus be used to control haemorrhage only if immediate delivery is to occur. Treatment of disseminated intravascular clotting and secondary hyperfibrinolysis (called *consumption coagulopathy*) with products such as heparin and fibrinolysis inhibitors (for example, aminocaproic acid (Epsikapron) or aprotinin (Trasylol)) may appear to have a rational basis, but the most careful supervision and control by laboratory studies under the care of a consultant haematologist would be essential. Fresh whole blood is the best fluid to give and fresh-frozen plasma may be used to provide clotting factors.

Method of delivery in cases of antepartum haemorrhage
If, as in most cases of severe concealed haemorrhage, the fetus is dead, vaginal delivery is usually accomplished with assistance in the second stage if necessary. Caesarean section may be indicated in cases of mixed accidental APH where the fetus has survived and vaginal delivery cannot be accomplished quickly.

UNAVOIDABLE ANTEPARTUM HAEMORRHAGE
Placenta praevia occurs in under 1% of all pregnancies and in all gravida groups. There is, however, an increased incidence in women who have had several pregnancies in rapid succession. Why this should occur is uncertain and the theory that the fertilized ovum implants itself low in the uterine cavity because chronic endometritis is associated with a smooth atrophic mucosa does not seem very reliable. Other theories postulate that low implantation is due to late development of the trophoblast or that the placenta is formed in the decidua

capsularis and not in the decidua basalis as is usual. The true aetiological factors involved remain unestablished.

Symptoms and degrees of placenta praevia

The only symptom of placenta praevia is vaginal haemorrhage. By definition this occurs after the 28th week of pregnancy and before the birth of the baby, but cases occurring earlier in pregnancy and diagnosed as threatened abortion may prove to be associated with placenta praevia. Furthermore, minor degrees of the condition may be missed, as bleeding may not take place until labour commences when the midwife considers the patient has had a heavy 'show'.

Four degrees of placenta praevia are defined:

(1)   The lower edge of the placenta just dips down into the lower segment (Figure 46(a)).
(2)   The lower edge reaches the internal os (Figure 46(b)).
(3)   The placenta covers the internal os when the latter is closed (Figure 46(c)).
(4)   The placenta lies centrally over the internal os and would cover the cervix even if fully dilated (assuming that the patient would survive to reach the second stage of labour) (Figure 46(d)).

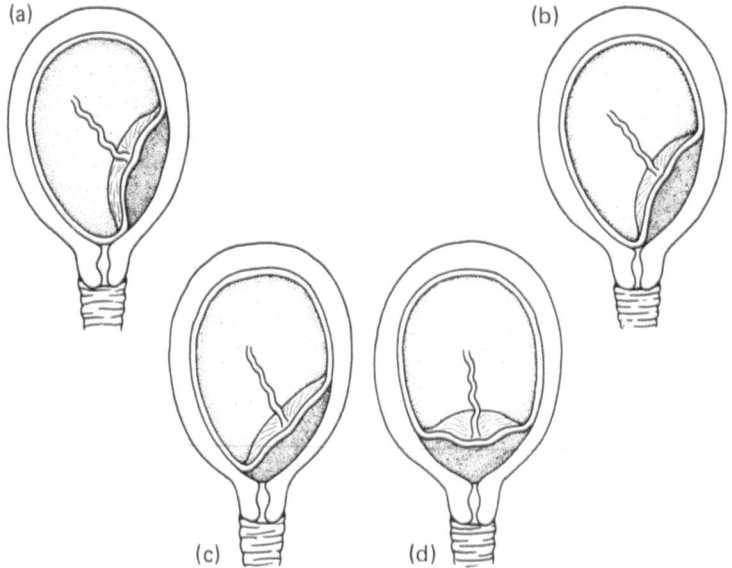

Figure 46   The types of placenta praevia. (a) First degree, (b) second degree, (c) third degree, (d) fourth degree

There are four words to describe the bleeding which typifies that associated with placenta praevia. These are:

Sudden
Painless
Causeless
Recurrent.

The '*warning haemorrhage*' is an excellent term used to describe the initial bleed of placenta praevia which is often slight. A red blood loss occurs suddenly and without warning. The patient may be in bed, sitting or walking about, and she will often say that she suddenly 'felt damp below'. She may think she has leaked urine but to her dismay finds that the loss is one of blood. Haemorrhage is sudden and completely painless with no prior discomfort or backache. This bleed is a 'warning' to the patient and her attendants who must immediately consider the diagnosis of placenta praevia.

It is, or course, possible that the initial bleed may be very severe indeed, but the majority of cases seen personally have had a 'warning haemorrhage' that in no way endangered life. Bleeding tends to be somewhat heavier and occur earlier in pregnancy when associated with the more serious degrees of placenta praevia.

The word 'causeless' indicates two features. There is no history of trauma (coitus, however, may precipitate the loss) and there is no associated toxaemia. The latter, a common complication of any pregnancy, may conceivably also be present, but it is a surprisingly rare association. Vaginal bleeding in placenta praevia will recur, and each subsequent loss tends to be heavier than the previous one.

Examination
Examination of the abdomen reveals no tenderness (there is no concealed haemorrhage) and the fetus is easily felt. Malpresentations are common and if the lie is longitudinal the presenting part is not engaged.

The features already described are but presumptive evidence pointing to the diagnosis of unavoidable APH, but the exact location of the placental site as yet remains unestablished. The best and most commonly used method to localize this site is by ultrasonic scanning to produce an echogram. With the necessary apparatus and an expert operator, placentography by this method may show not only the relationship of the placenta to the cervix, but also its thickness and whether it is anteriorly or posteriorly situated.

Other methods used to determine the placental site include:

(1)   Injection of radioactive isotopes, after which the abdomen is scanned with a scintillation counter. High readings indicate the position of the placenta.

(2)   Soft tissue radiography. This has been replaced more or less by ultrasonic scanning which is more accurate.

(3)   Arteriography and thermography have also been used.

If facilities for placentography are not available, the only method for determining definitely whether or not the placenta is situated in the lower segment is to explore the latter digitally. *The fact that in no circumstances should a vaginal examination be attempted when placenta praevia is considered possible cannot be overstressed.* If the placenta is touched, even lightly, resultant haemorrhage may be so profuse that the outcome could be fatal if adequate facilities for treatment are not immediately available. Thus, vaginal examination in cases of suspected placenta praevia may be performed only in hospital with the patient under anaesthesia and all facilities for immediate caesarean section present.

Treatment

During the Second World War, maternal mortality associated with placenta praevia in the United Kingdom dropped 10-fold (from about 6−0.6%). This was due partly to improved facilities for blood transfusion and to the discovery of the rhesus factor and antibiotics. However, the main reason for this dramatic fall was the recognition that treatment must be expectant, in other words no vaginal examination (rectal is even more dangerous), and no vaginal packs. Expectant treatment involves immediate transfer of the patient to hospital where she will remain and where crossmatched blood is always held ready. Bedrest for several days with no fresh bleeding is essential, and although the patient may then be allowed out of bed, she must remain in hospital as long as placenta praevia is considered a possibility. Sedation may be indicated.

No patient will die in hospital from haemorrhage if adequate blood replacement is available. The aim now is to allow the pregnancy to continue to its final month when the chances of fetal survival are high, with delivery at about the 38th week. The patient is transferred to the operating theatre for examination under anaesthesia (EUA) and possible caesarean section. EUA is unnecessary if the exact siting of the placenta is known, and in the days before placentography I often dispensed with EUA when clinically a major degree of placenta praevia was judged likely.

Delivery is effected by artificial rupture of the membranes in cases of first-degree placenta praevia and by caesarean section for all other grades. Some may consider amniotomy for anteriorly situated second-degree placenta praevia as pressure by the fetal head on the venous sinuses may stop further haemorrhage.

Perinatal mortality which was approximately 50% in 1939 dropped to about 15% in 1945 and is now under 5% in many areas. Maternal mortality associated with placenta praevia in England and Wales is now about 0.1%.

A patient with suspected placenta praevia must not be allowed to progress to the first stage of labour without active measures being taken. If labour cannot be stopped and the pregnancy has not reached the 36th week, it may be necessary to initiate the above management forthwith.

18

Contracted pelvis and disproportion

A contracted pelvis is one in which either the shape or size is sufficiently abnormal to cause difficulty in the delivery of a normal-sized fetus. *Disproportion* is a term which embraces a wider group and indicates any disparity in size between the fetus and pelvis that will lead to difficulties in labour, or *dystocia*. Thus, even when the patient has a normal pelvis, disproportion will exist if the fetus presents by the brow, has hydrocephalus or is excessively large. A badly flexed occipito-posterior position may also cause disproportion.

Types of pelvis
In the description of the bony pelvis in Chapter 1 it was stated that for the purpose of obstetrics the true pelvis only was of significance, and that the splayed-out portion of the ilium which constitutes the false pelvis could be ignored. Broad or narrow hips, size of feet or shoes and height of patient assume little importance in indicating the capacity of a woman's pelvis when compared with clinical estimation (but see remarks on stature below). The three areas of the true pelvis to consider in every case are the inlet or brim, the cavity and the outlet. The capacity of the inlet depends upon both its shape and measurements, while that of the cavity will be determined to a large extent by the contour of the anterior surface of the sacrum, the prominence of the ischial spines and whether or not the side walls converge. The more important part of the pelvic outlet to assess is the anterior half or subpubic arch, so the subpubic angle and intertuberous diameter are significant.

Human pelves have been typed in different ways, but a classification made by Caldwell and Mulloy remains the best. There is, however, much overlap within the groups and features of any pelvis may have characteristics of more than one type. The four main groups of pelves are gynaecoid, android, platypelloid, and anthropoid (Figure 47).

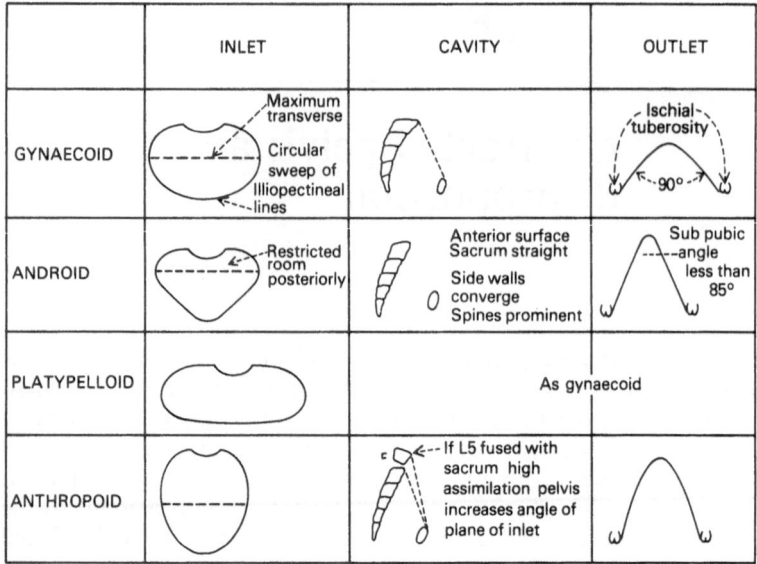

	INLET	CAVITY	OUTLET
GYNAECOID	Maximum transverse — Circular sweep of Illiopectineal lines		Ischial tuberosity — 90°
ANDROID	Restricted room posteriorly	Anterior surface Sacrum straight — Side walls converge — Spines prominent	Sub pubic angle less than 85°
PLATYPELLOID		As gynaecoid	
ANTHROPOID		If L5 fused with sacrum high assimilation pelvis increases angle of plane of inlet	

Figure 47 Characteristics of the four types of pelves

GYNAECOID PELVIS

The normal female pelvis is gynaecoid in type and best adapted for childbirth. It has been described above (page 3). Basically the gynaecoid pelvis is round, shallow and roomy. The inlet is round, the anterior surface of the sacrum shows a shallow concavity, the side walls do not converge, the ischial spines are not prominent and the subpubic angle approaches 90°.

ANDROID PELVIS

This type of pelvis is normally found in the male. The inlet space is reduced as the maximum transverse diameter tends to lie posteriorly and the anterior portion is triangular in shape. The side walls of the pelvis are convergent, the ischial spines prominent and the front of the sacrum is straight. The subpubic angle is less than 85° which makes it more difficult for the fetal head to pivot out. With this type of pelvis, the head tends to enter the brim imperfectly flexed and there may be deep transverse arrest (page 92).

PLATYPELLOID PELVIS

This is the simple flat pelvis in which the transverse diameter of the pelvic inlet is long and the antero-posterior diameter is short. The pelvic cavity and outlet are often normal (that is, gynaecoid), and even though the true conjugate diameter is reduced, spontaneous vaginal delivery is common. The head tends to enter the pelvis to one side and inclines to one or other of the shoulders (*asynclitism*) so that the reduced space in the inlet is fully utilized.

ANTHROPOID PELVIS
This type of pelvis found in the anthropoid apes has a pelvic inlet with a long antero-posterior and a short transverse diameter. The sacral surface is straight and may be elongated because the last lumbar vertebra is fused with it. This sacralization of the fifth lumbar vertebra (or *high assimilation* pelvis), gives a false sacral promontory and increases the angle of the pelvic inlet (see Figure 47). The subpubic angle tends to be reduced.

The anthropoid pelvis is not uncommon (under 10%) and persistent occipito-posterior positions with face-to-pubis delivery may occur. The posterior part of the inlet is more roomy and accommodates the occiput more readily.

Other types of contracted pelvis include:

(1) The generally contracted pelvis which is a small gynaecoid pelvis with all measurements reduced. It is also known as a *justominor* pelvis.
(2) Contracted outlet. The pelvic inlet is normal but the pelvis is 'funnel'-shaped; this is uncommon.
(3) Asymmetrical pelves which may result from a variety of causes including fractures, spinal diseases and curvature, and congenital bony pelvic abnormalities. (Nägele and Robert described pelves such as these about 140 years ago!).
(4) Pelves altered by bony diseases such as rickets (rachitic flat pelvis) or osteomalacia (very rarely seen in the United Kingdom).

These and other types of contracted pelves require individual consideration by the obstetrician and specialist colleagues to decide how best to manage pregnancy, delivery and thereafter.

Diagnosis of contracted pelvis and disproportion
Features of importance are as follows.

OBSTETRIC HISTORY
If a patient has had a spontaneous delivery of a child weighing 3500 g or more with no difficulty, and the child is alive and well, it is reasonable to assume that her pelvis is adequate. It must be remembered, however, that subsequent births tend to result in heavier babies and that the degree of flexion of the head in cephalic presentations is

important. A woman with a previous history of a difficult forceps extraction associated possibly with maternal and/or fetal damage should be most carefully assessed and all reasons for possible cephalo-pelvic disproportion at her previous pregnancy considered.

APPEARANCE AND TYPE OF THE PATIENT
The 'gynaecoid' woman with normal secondary sex characteristics, normal menstrual pattern and fertility is more likely to have a gynae-coid pelvis than a woman with very marked male attributes. The latter may have scanty, infrequent periods and have had difficulty in becom-ing pregnant. *Hirsutism* in the female is a common deviation from normal secondary sex characteristics and more often than not is a con-stitutional feature of no significance. Many women have a male type distribution of pubic hair which rises to the umbilicus in a triangular fashion instead of terminating suprapubically in a horizontal line.

The short adipose patient, especially with a girdle distribution of fat, may have a long labour with poor uterine contractions, and the term *dystrophia dystocia syndrome* is sometimes used to describe this condition.

MALPRESENTATIONS AND THE 'PENDULOUS' BELLY
These should alert the examiner to possible disproportion.

NON-ENGAGEMENT OF THE HEAD
Non-engagement of the head in a primigravida by the 38th week of pregnancy is commonly due to an occipito-posterior position assoc-iated with incomplete flexion of the head, although often no obvious cause is found. In certain African races it is usual to find that the fetal

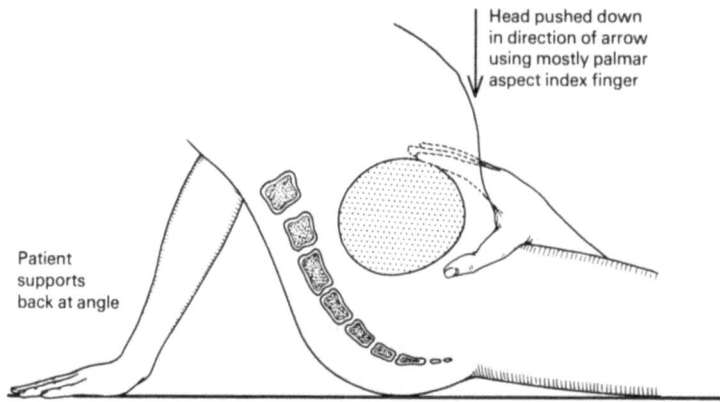

Figure 48   Method of 'pushing' head into pelvis to eliminate diagnosis of disproportion

head does not descend into the pelvis until the second stage of labour has been reached. This is probably due to racial differences in the tilt of the pelvic inlet.

If the fetal head can be made to engage in the pelvis and the outlet is clinically adequate, disproportion may be excluded. A good method by which this may be attempted is to ask the patient to sit up and to support herself with arms outstretched behind her, resting palms comfortably on the couch. The plane of the pelvic inlet is almost horizontal when her back is at an angle of just below 45°. The practitioner adds support to the patient's back with the left hand and pushes the head down vertically into the pelvis using the radial aspect of the right palm. The patient must be informed of the manoeuvre and the reason for it, and the pressure must be gently but not tentatively applied and sustained (Figure 48). This should cause no discomfort.

An alternative test which does not involve pressure, is shown in Figure 49. Here the index finger is placed on the symphysis pubis while the fingertips of the other hand slide over the head in the direction shown, that is at right angles to the plane of the inlet. If the fingertips pass well under the finger on the pubis, there is no anterior overlap of the head. Allowance is made for the thickness of the pubic bone.

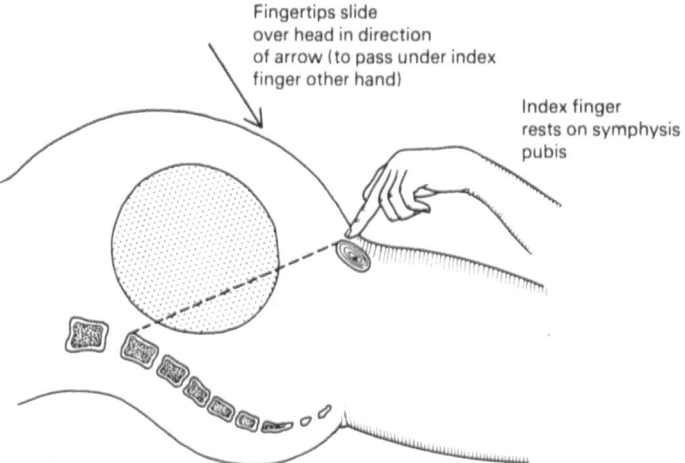

Fingertips slide
over head in direction
of arrow (to pass under index
finger other hand)

Index finger
rests on symphysis
pubis

Figure 49   Testing for anterior overlap of the head

PELVIC MEASUREMENTS

Clinical examination of the true pelvis is most important and has been discussed above (page 5). A vaginal examination with two fingers assesses the pelvic cavity, and external pelvimetry is reserved solely for an estimate of the capacity of the pelvic outlet.

X-RAY PELVIMETRY

A standing lateral pelvimetry picture should be taken in all cases of suspected disproportion and can give the obstetrician much clinical information. The patient must be correctly positioned and the X-ray is best taken in very late pregnancy or in early labour. The precise measurement of the anterior-posterior diameter of the inlet (true conjugate) is obtained as well as those of the mid-cavity and outlet. The curve of the anterior surface of the sacrum is important and in the gynaecoid pelvis should be gently concave. The sacrosciatic or greater sciatic notch leading to the ischial spines should be shallow, and if combined with a normal sacrum will indicate a pelvic cavity which is not too deep. A deep pelvic cavity might contribute to dystocia.

The fetal skull is seen and its maximum diameter may be compared with the true conjugate diameter of the pelvis. If the fetal head is high, two pencil lines on the X-ray plate may be drawn at right angles from either end of the inlet antero-posterior diameter to project it as shown in Figure 50 and facilitate cephalo-pelvic comparison. Overlap of the fetal skull bones may suggest pressure, and excessive moulding indicates disproportion. Although one usually cannot be certain from a lateral picture which prominence of the skull is the occiput, the fetal spine prior to labour is not twisted. So the fetal vertebrae will indicate

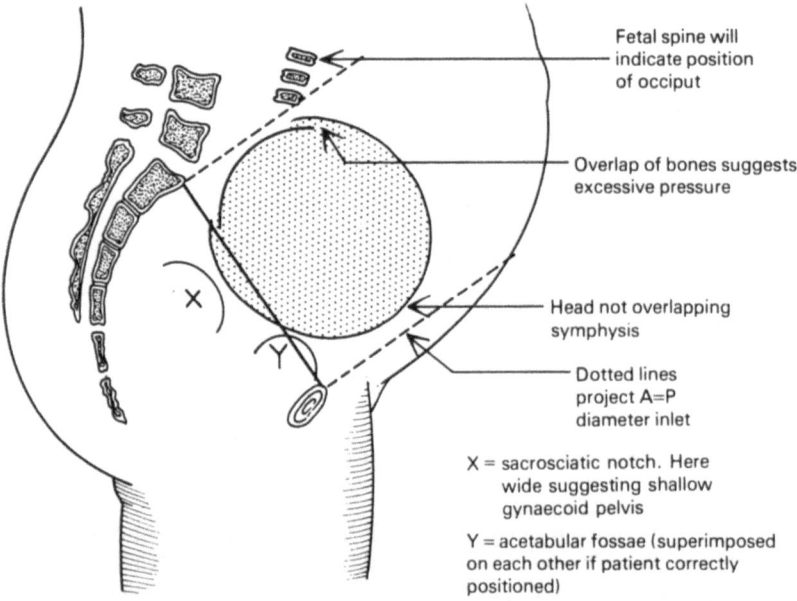

Fetal spine will indicate position of occiput

Overlap of bones suggests excessive pressure

Head not overlapping symphysis

Dotted lines project A=P diameter inlet

X = sacrosciatic notch. Here wide suggesting shallow gynaecoid pelvis

Y = acetabular fossae (superimposed on each other if patient correctly positioned)

Figure 50   The features of a lateral X-ray pelvimetry film

the position of the occiput – in other words, if the fetal spine is adjacent to the maternal spine the occiput is posterior.

An X-ray film of the pelvic inlet is not usually taken in pregnancy as it requires more radiation. If necessary, this may be taken after delivery to help management in a subsequent pregnancy. A pelvic outlet view usually adds very little information to the clinical picture.

Management of disproportion and trial of labour

The management of labour in cases of suspected disproportion may be by one of four methods.

(1) *Trial of labour* – see below.

(2) *Caesarean section.* This is indicated when

(a) disproportion is absolute, for example when the true conjugate diameter measures 9 cm or less;

(b) the patient is an elderly primigravida. The question that now arises is 'how old is an elderly primigravida?' and it is difficult to answer this simply and numerically. Although statistics indicate that a woman over 25 years of age has a longer labour on average than a patient aged 18, factors such as social conditions, general build and the time taken to become pregnant may also be significant. A woman of 30 years of age is entering this category and has certainly arrived by her 35th birthday! (Be gentle in the use of the term 'elderly'. Lack of oestrogens after the menopause may cause atrophic vaginitis, too often called 'senile vaginitis'. I have met many women of 40 or thereabouts who were justifiably irate because they were told they had senile vaginitis!)

(c) a breech presentation is associated with a contracted pelvis;

(d) other obstetric or medical complications are present, for example pre-eclampsia.

(3) *Induction of premature labour.* This may be considered in multiparae with a history of maternal and/or fetal complications following vaginal delivery of a large baby.

(4) *Symphysiotomy.* This is not often performed in United Kingdom. The symphysis pubis is cut through, usually with a scalpel, carefully guarding the urethra. The capacity of the pelvis is increased only very slightly and the severed joint may possibly become a site of pain in later years. Caesarean section is preferred by most obstetricians.

Destructive operations on a living fetus should rarely be performed for disproportion and would indicate mismanagement rather than management.

Trial of labour

There are some features in labour that cannot be forecast with certainty and thus the patient may be given a 'trial of labour'. The uncertainties include.

(1)   The strength and nature of the uterine contractions.
(2)   The amount of moulding the fetal head will undergo with safety.
(3)   The degree of flexion that will occur (in an occipito-posterior position).
(4)   The degree of 'give' or stretching of the maternal pelvis during the passage of the head.

The idea behind a so-called trial is to watch carefully the effect of labour (that is, of myometrial contraction and retraction) on the descent of the fetal head and the dilatation of the cervix. As long as both maternal and fetal conditions remain satisfactory, the cervix continues to dilate progressively and the head to descend, and safe vaginal delivery remains likely, the trial may continue. If at any time in the first stage of labour maternal or fetal distress becomes manifest, immediate delivery by caesarean section is indicated. The latter would also be performed if it became apparent that safe vaginal delivery is unlikely, a decision that normally will be made within 24 hours of the onset of labour.

Many today consider, justifiably, that with ideal conditions there is no difference between a trial of labour and any other labour. Every mother and baby is watched with care during labour which may be said to be normal only in retrospect. A generation ago, if a patient underwent a trial of labour vaginal examinations were kept to a minimum to reduce the risk of introducing infection, especially as caesarean section was a more likely outcome. (Rectal examinations which were performed to estimate cervical dilatation and station of the head carried an even greater risk of introducing infection.) This restriction on vaginal examinations is now not applicable as aseptic and antiseptic techniques have advanced considerably, and indeed such examinations are essential at least at the onset of labour and when the membranes rupture to exclude cord complications.

The term a 'trial of labour' is still widely used to establish the regime of management. It is conducted almost invariably in a primigravida with a fetus whose head is not engaged at the onset of labour and where a minor degree of disproportion is considered possible. Such a labour would necessarily be in a hospital, preferably with monitoring facilities. Information available should include a lateral pelvimetry film.

The disadvantages of a trial of labour are that the patient may undergo a long labour which predisposes to postpartum haemorrhage and increases the risk of infection. Furthermore, long labour may be terminated by the patient requiring caesarean section.

The risks to the fetus include premature rupture of the membranes and prolapsed cord, and there is the danger that excessive moulding may cause intracranial damage.

The advantages of a trial of labour are that labour is usually not induced and thus the baby will not be born prematurely. Furthermore, if labour is terminated by caesarean section the indications for abdominal delivery will have been definitely established.

19

Abnormal uterine action

The arrangement of the three layers of muscle fibres of the uterus in late pregnancy and labour has been described in Chapter 7. The layers are not as clearly defined as shown diagrammatically in Figure 51, but the fibres in general thin out as they approach the uterine isthmus and cervix. The waves of contraction and retraction which commence in the area of the cornua become less intense as they pass downwards to the lower segment. As the latter has a higher percentage of circular muscle fibres than the fundus it has been aptly

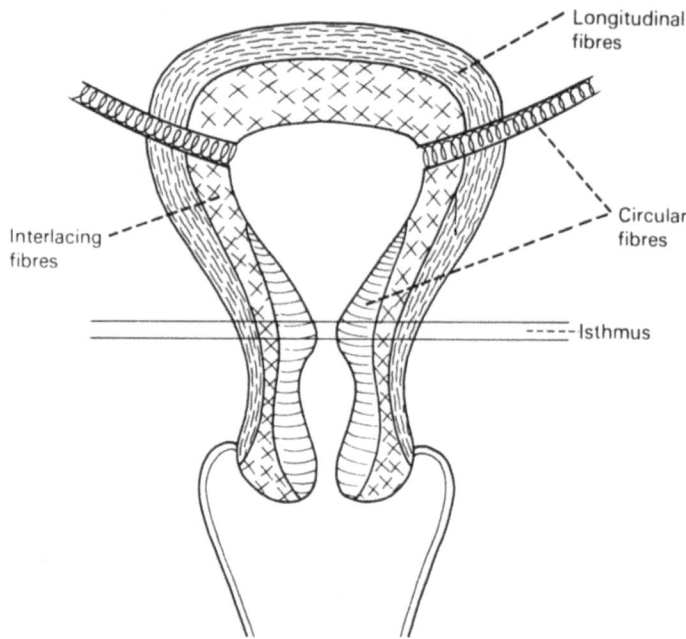

Figure 51   Arrangement of uterine muscle fibres during labour

compared to a sphincter which may go into spasm through fear stimulating the sympathetic nervous system. Yet the lower segment needs to remain passive and relaxed in order to efface and dilate, and any effort to do so if in spasm would cause pain. Pain increases fear and thus a vicious circle is set up which must be broken if normal labour is to occur. These views, much debated years ago, may be oversimplistic, but even today the innervation of the uterus in labour is neither fully established nor understood. The pathways by which fibres of the autonomic nervous system reach the uterus may be agreed, but the physiological effects of stimuli remain unestablished. Alpha (a) and beta (β)-receptor sites in the myometrium have been noted (page 74) but the entire picture of myometrial activity is complicated by hormonal influences. Indeed, even in the non-pregnant state, uterine responses to hormonal influences may differ according to the time of the menstrual cycle.

It is not surprising therefore, that variations in the classification of abnormal uterine action are numerous and sometimes lead to confusion.

There are basically two groups of abnormal uterine action that may cause dystocia. The resting uterine muscle tone may be poor (*hypotonic*) and result in feeble or no contractions, or the muscle tone may be high (*hypertonic*). A hypertonic upper segment may contract spasmodically and not work in harmony with the lower segment. Older terms such as 'colicky uterus' and 'disordered polarity' were apt descriptions. These states are discussed below.

Hypotonic uterine inertia
Myometrial activity may be poor from the onset of labour, or initially may be normal or excessive and then diminish as 'uterine exhaustion' becomes manifest. Thus primary and secondary hypotonic uterine states are distinguished.

PRIMARY HYPOTONIC INERTIA
The causes of this state are:

(1) Poor muscle tone due to
  (a) Overdistension of the uterus associated with conditions such as hydramnios or twin pregnancy.
  (b) Grandmultiparity.
  (c) Fibroids.
  (d) Maternal malnutrition and/or anaemia.
  (e) Hormonal defects. The defect may possibly be a deficiency of oestrogen or of oxytocin from the posterior pituitary

gland; or inadequate amounts of prostaglandin may be synthesized and released by the decidua. It is possible, too, that there could be an intrinsic defect in the muscle cell itself (perhaps at the receptor sites). In practical terms under this heading are included the cases of hypotonic inertia for which no obvious cause is found. Fear or other emotional upsets may be associated with poor uterine action, an altered hormone status being due to the effect on the hypothalamus which is influenced by the higher centres of the brain.

(2)   A full bladder and/or rectum can inhibit contractions.

(3)   An ill-fitting presenting part as in malpresentations and cases of disproportion, or where the head remains high for any reason. A badly flexed occipito-posterior position is not uncommonly found. The presenting part that is well applied to the cervix undoubtedly promotes normal uterine contractions, probably by a stimulating effect on the nerve plexuses and promoting the release of oxytocin.

Treatment

The important points in the treatment of primary hypotonic uterine inertia are to maintain the patient's morale and ensure that she has adequate rest with the correct administration of sedatives if and when required (oversedation too early may be a causative factor). However, if labour has not been fully established and there is no obvious contra-indication, the patient may prefer to be up and about. Dehydration and acetoketosis are avoided as described under management of the first stage of labour (Chapter 9). The first stage may be managed actively with intravenous oxytocic infusion (page 96), provided no disproportion exists, and artificial rupture of the membranes if there is no evidence of presentation of the cord.

SECONDARY HYPOTONIC INERTIA

In this condition labour may have been proceeding quite normally for some hours, then contractions weaken in intensity and become less frequent and eventually may cease altogether. The condition occurs at any stage and not uncommonly in the second stage of labour when a minor degree of disproportion and/or a rigid pelvic floor may be responsible.

Treatment will depend upon the stage of labour in which the hypotonic state occurs and the cause. This could entail sedation, oxytocic infusion, ventouse extraction or, if the cervix has reached full dilatation, forceps extraction, and/or episiotomy.

Caesarean section may occasionally be necessary, but although always preferable to a difficult vaginal delivery it is not usually indicated as treatment for hypotonic uterine inertia in the absence of other obstetric complications.

The rigid cervix or cervical dystocia

In this condition, a cause of delay in the first stage of labour, there is no progressive dilatation of the cervix in spite of good uterine contractions. Organic rigidity of the cervix may be responsible, but this is not common. Possible causes for this are cervical fibroids, previous operations (such as cone biopsy, amputation at prolapse repair, or trachelorrhaphy) and, rarely, carcinoma of the cervix. Cervical dystocia is more commonly associated with what is best described as a functional failure of the cervix to relax, a condition that occurs in the hypertonic states described below.

Treatment

Sedation may suffice but if organic rigidity is present caesarean section will be indicated. Small incisions of the cervix (Dührssen) and made in positions corresponding to 2, 6 and 10 hours on the clock are sometimes used prior to forceps extraction, but the risk of extension of the incisions and haemorrhage is high and most obstetricians in the United Kingdom prefer to deliver the baby abdominally.

The hypertonic uterus or incoordinate uterine action

Hypertonic uterine action is associated with a uterus that has a high resting muscle tone. Strong spasmodic and painful contractions occur, yet there is no advance in the first stage of labour. The patient experiences abdominal pain and backache before the contraction can be felt by palpation, and pain continues after the contraction has passed. Eventually the pain may become incessant and the uterus pass into spasm (*tonic contraction*) applying itself tightly to fetus and placenta, and by obstructing the blood flow through the latter cause anoxic conditions and fetal death.

Intensive studies of the behaviour of cells of the myometrium in labour continue. They include electronmicroscopy, studies of biochemical and electrical activity and recordings of intrauterine and intra-myometrial pressures. A picture of the activity of contraction and the unique phenomenon of retraction is thus built up. A descending gradient of activity is described which normally weakens considerably as it passes from fundus to cervix. This is not surprising as the muscle component of the cervix is very much less. The pattern of spread of activity, it is stated, may pass from isthmus upwards to fundus and downwards to the cervix, thus accounting for cervical dystocia in the absence of organic cause. Patterns are entirely absent in the 'colicky uterus' where segments of muscle contract and retract independently. Clinically, however, these conditions in which a hypertonic uterus exhibits incoordinate action are similar.

CONTRACTION OR CONSTRICTION RING DYSTOCIA

This is also a type of hypertonic action associated with spasm of circular muscle fibres, which can occur in any stage of labour but is rare in the first stage. In the second stage of labour delay will occur and the ring is diagnosed when felt on internal examination. It often forms around a depression such as the fetal neck. An *'hour glass' contraction ring* in the third stage of labour is the most common manifestation of this type of abnormal uterine action (page 78).

CAUSES OF HYPERTONIC UTERINE ACTION

These are:

(1) Hormonal or intrinsic defect in muscle cell. The comments made under the heading 1(e) above (page 177) are applicable (in reverse) and incoordinate hypertonic uterine action is found with no apparent cause. Fear and emotional factors are again factors.

(2) Malpresentations and disproportion can cause any type of abnormal uterine action.

(3) Uterine manipulations such as external cephalic version in early labour, and excessive handling during the management of the third stage may increase muscular irritability.

(4) The injudicious use of oxytocic drugs also increases muscular irritability. When an oxytocic drug is used in the first and second stages of labour, intravenous administration is best. Other routes such as intramuscular, oral, nasal ('pitocin snuff') intrauterine and intravaginal (prostaglandin pessaries) have all been used, but dosage control is must less effective. An oxytocic infusion should be commenced with a dilute solution (5 units/litre oxytocin) given slowly initially, 10 drops per minute or less, and preferably used with an infusion pump.

Treatment

All avoidable causative factors should be borne in mind. Sedation to diminish the activity of the hypertonic uterus with incoordinate action also has the effect of reducing fear and pain. The value of epidural analgesia in this respect has been mentioned (page 100) and is most useful. Otherwise oxytocic administration, if being given, should stop, and sedation intramuscularly with, say, pethidine and promazine may be administered. Intravenous drip transfusion of the latter two drugs in 5% glucose, or diazepam therapy are also used (page 99).

A contraction ring causing delay in the second stage of labour, or retained placenta in the third stage, is treated by administering general anaesthesia until the spasm disappears when the fetus may be extracted with forceps or the placenta removed manually.

Obstructed labour and rupture of the uterus

Labour, once established, will continue until the baby is expelled. It may be possible, temporarily, to halt the progress of labour, but eventual expulsion of the baby from the uterus is inevitable. If vaginal delivery is impossible, the baby must be born via the uterine wall, and the only safe method of achieving this is by caesarean section. If the latter is not performed in time, the baby will be expelled into the abdominal cavity by rupture of the uterus. Except in very rare cases the baby will not survive and it will be essential to take immediate resuscitative and operative measures to save the mother's life. Rupture of the uterus may rarely take place without warning – the so-called silent rupture – although tenderness over the site of a previous uterine scar suggests that this might happen and will alert the practitioner. Obstructed labour leading to ruptured uterus should never occur if there is adequate supervision of the patient. The causes of obstructed labour are absolute disproportion including cases of brow and shoulder presentations and persistent mento-posterior positions, fetal abnormalities such as hydrocephalus, and the presence of pelvic tumours. The deflexed occipito-posterior position especially when associated with a contracted pelvis must also be considered.

Before the uterus ruptures in obstructed labour the following sequence of events occurs.

(1) Periods of uterine activity alternate with periods of hypotonic inertia. During each period of activity the upper segment of the uterus thickens and becomes smaller, while the lower segment thins and is pulled up.

(2) Eventually a *pathological retraction ring*, or *ring of Bandl*, forms where the very thick upper segment meets the high and very thin lower segment. Bandl's ring can be seen and felt through the abdominal wall.

(3) The upper segment goes into spasm, (*generalized tonic contraction*).

(4) Rupture of the lower segment follows (3) above.

CLINICAL FEATURES
As stated above, periods of uterine activity alternate with periods of 'uterine exhaustion'. Maternal exhaustion, too, is manifest and the patient becomes restless and may vomit. Pulse rate and temperature rise, and dehydration becomes evident although the patient's skin may be cold and moist instead of hot and dry. Urine analysis shows protein, acetone and even blood to be present. Abdominal pain is severe and eventually becomes constant. The depression of Bandl's ring, which can be seen and felt, will rise to a higher level in the abdominal wall and is a sign that immediate action is essential to avoid uterine rupture. The occurrence of the latter is accompanied by profound shock even though the severe pain the patient has suffered may be dramatically relieved as uterine contractions cease.

Treatment of obstructed labour
Immediate caesarean section must be performed, and uterine activity must be diminished or stopped while preparations for surgery are made. Intravenous sedation may do this, but the administration of a general anaesthetic is better. The patient, lying on her left side, should be given the maximum amounts of oxygen by the anaesthetist. If intravenous sedation has been used, pure oxygen through a nasal mask may be administered.

    Lower segment caesarean section is the treatment of choice even if the fetus is dead. Destructive operations (such as craniotomy) may be performed in some areas, but the maternal risk is high as Bandl's ring indicates that the lower segment is very thin indeed and may thus rupture during attempts at vaginal delivery. The comparative risks to the mother of abdominal and vaginal delivery of a dead fetus must be carefully considered by the obstetrician.

20

The placenta and its functions: maturity and the at-risk fetus

The placenta, the structure through which maternal–fetal exchanges take place, has several other important functions. The well-being of the fetus depends upon it receiving an adequate supply of oxygen and nutrients, and to achieve this it is essential that the flow and composition of the maternal blood reaching the placenta is normal, that the amount of healthy functioning placental tissue is adequate, and that the fetus itself is normal and able to utilize properly the supplies received and to eliminate waste products. Maternal–fetal exchanges occur through the chorionic villi where the bloodstreams of the mother and baby are separated by the fetal capillary endothelium, connective tissue of the mesoderm and trophoblast (see page 31). Exchanges take place either by diffusion or more active processes in which cells ingest surrounding fluid (*pinocytosis*). Experts in the field of placental function and research consider that the term 'placental insufficiency' as the cause of fetal deprivation should be avoided, as faults in the maternal supply line to the placenta are usually factors of more significance (Gruenwald, 1975)*.

Important functions of the placenta
The placenta has six vital functions:

(1) *Respiratory*. The gaseous exchange of oxygen from mother to fetus, and carbon dioxide in the reverse direction, takes place by simple diffusion between the two blood circulations.
(2) *Nutritive*. Glucose, amino acids (for protein synthesis), lipids (especially free fatty acids), vitamins, electrolytes and minerals such as iron, calcium and magnesium are among the nutrients transferred to the fetus.

*Gruenwald, P. (1975). *The Placenta*. (Lancaster: MTP Press).

(3) *Excretory.* In addition to carbon dioxide mentioned above, waste products such as urea are discharged into the maternal circulation and are excreted by the mother.

(4) *Barrier.* Many, but not all, organisms are unable to pass through the placenta. The spirochoete of syphilis can do so as can many viruses, the most notable being rubella. The barrier action of the placenta, generally most effective, is not always perfect, and it is known for example that fetal red blood cells occasionally enter the maternal circulation. This is important with regard to conditions such as erythroblastosis fetalis. Some antibodies, too, may cross the placental barrier although most with a potent cytotoxic action cannot (usually of the IgM type − macroimmunoglobulin). The smaller molecule, IgG gammaglobulin, can pass through the placenta, and the antibodies or haemagglutinins made by the mother in Rh, ABO and other fetal − maternal red cell incompatibilities are of this type (see page 230).

(5) *Immunological.* In addition to the defence provided by passive transfer of some antibodies from the mother, the placenta protects the fetus from undergoing immunological rejection by the mother with whom the fetus is histoincompatible.

(6) *Hormonal.* The placenta synthesizes oestrogens, progesterone, chorionic gonadotrophin (HCG) and chorionic somatomammmotrophin (HCS). Many other polypeptide hormones have been found in placental extracts but it is uncertain whether or not they have been synthesized by the placenta. Of particular interest is *relaxin* which is believed to relax the joints of the body.

Prematurity and dysmaturity
Over the past decade increasing stress has been placed on the importance of differentiating between the small infant born 'prematurely' and the small, so-called *'dysmature'* infant. The term 'prematurity', originally applied internationally to the condition of any infant whose birthweight was 2500 g or less is no longer used. If the pregnancy has not reached the end of the 37th week when the baby is delivered, the expression *'preterm'* infant is to be preferred. Infants may be smaller than normal for their gestational age because they have been deprived of the essentials for normal growth for reasons as discussed in the opening paragraph of this chapter. Terms applied to these infants are:

(1) Small (or light)-for-dates babies (SFD).
(2) Intrauterine growth retardation.
(3) Dysmaturity. (Although babies of diabetic mothers are larger than normal, the infants are usually lethargic initially and prone to

hypoglycaemia and respiratory distress; they, too, are at high risk and may be described as being dysmature).

It is, of course, not always possible to state accurately the duration of a pregnancy and this subject with causes for error in estimating the date of delivery has been discussed in Chapter 3. For many reasons pregnancy may require termination by induction of labour or caesarean section (page 194) and often the indications for intervention are associated with related causes of intrauterine growth retardation. Fetal survival may be jeopardized if the timing for intervention is misjudged. These are problems which remain of the greatest importance although their solution is assisted by tests for placental efficiency, and estimations of intrauterine growth and fetal maturity. Perinatal mortality and morbidity will also be diminished by the detection of fetal distress at its onset, by monitoring the fetal condition and by delivery in centres with fully equipped special care neonatal units. As only a small percentage of women have access to such centres it is of importance to recognize 'high-risk' cases so that the best arrangements possible for the confinement are made in good time.

PRETERM DELIVERY
This may be associated with:

(1)   Pre-eclampsia and toxaemias (Chapter 14).
(2)   Antepartum haemorrhage (Chapter 17).
In both these conditions the fetus may also be affected by intrauterine growth retardation (see below) and induction of labour may be indicated.
(3)   Multiple pregnancy.
(4)   Fetal abnormalities, especially when associated with hydramnios.
(5)   Maternal pyrexia due to any cause.
(6)   Trauma. Direct injury is a rare cause as is external cephalic version when performed gently (page 109). Of interest, however, is an increased perinatal mortality in the United Kingdom and Eastern European countries associated with preterm births following the increased incidence of therapeutic abortion.
(7)   Developmental abnormalities of the uterus, or fibroids (page 150).
(8)   A previous history of abortion and/or preterm delivery.
(9)   No obvious cause is found in many cases. Sometimes premature rupture of the membranes may be due to an intrinsic weakness in the membranes themselves, or an incompetent internal os (a factor of possible significance following trauma (see (6) above).
(10)   Intervention by the obstetrician.

Unmarried women under the age of 18 appear to have an increased risk of preterm labour.

INTRAUTERINE GROWTH RETARDATION
In addition to the causes as specified above (especially (1), (2) and (3)) intrauterine growth retardation may be associated with:

(1)   Socioeconomic status, as both fetal deprivation and preterm delivery are more common in the lower socioeconomic groups.
(2)   Maternal conditions such as anaemia, malnutrition and certain heart conditions: also infections, especially rubella or cytomegalovirus (CMV).
(3)   Fetal malformations and genetic factors and abnormalities and diseases connected with isoimmunization.
(4)   Maternal age. Women over 35 are at increased risk.
(5)   Smoking during pregnancy. Nicotine affects maternal and fetal blood and a reported high concentration of carboxyhaemoglobin in both bloodstreams is probably responsible for dysmaturity. Chronic alcoholism and drug addiction may be related to maternal personality, lifestyle and nutrition, and associated with intrauterine fetal deprivation.
(6)   Racial and geographical differences. These are not wholly associated with socioeconomic factors (see (1) above), and statistical studies suggest that genetic influences play a part. In many developing countries lower average birthweights are normal and acceptable, and one often quoted example is that of a Malaysian baby whose average birthweight is almost 400 g lower than that of a European infant.
(7)   Placental influences. The placenta has a large reserve capacity as stated earlier, and because most placental changes are secondary to alterations in the maternal or fetal circulation through it, the term 'placental insufficiency' is condemned by some experts. However, placental infarction if extensive (as seen especially in hypertensive states) is associated with intrauterine growth retardation. Infarcts, often caused by thrombosis in the maternal spiral arterioles (page 33), appear as firm dark red wedge-shaped areas which become hard and white as the placenta ages. Furthermore, structural anomalies such as the *circumvallate placenta* may occasionally cause fetal deprivation. In this condition an elevated ridge-like fold which marks the transition from villous to membranous chorion is seen within the circumference of the fetal margin of the placenta. This is a form of placenta extrachorialis and the zone outside the ridge plays no part in the nutritive function of the placenta (Figure 52).

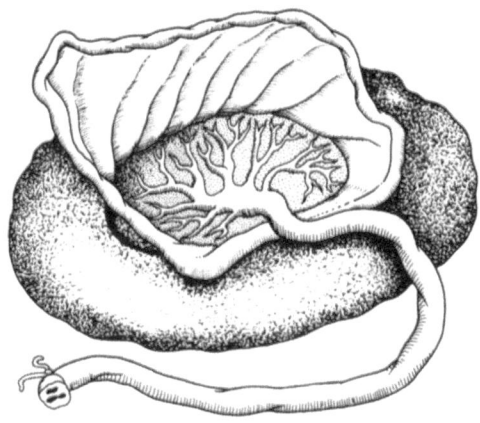

Figure 52   The circumvallate placenta

Prolonged pregnancy (postmaturity or post-term delivery)
It is generally accepted that prolonged pregnancy (postmaturity) *per se* constitutes a fetal hazard, although in the past the increased perinatal mortality has been ascribed to ordinary obstetric hazards such as dystocia and maternal hypertension. The most significant hazard, however, is that associated with the ageing of the placenta which becomes far less effective in nourishing and oxygenating the fetus; the rate of placental blood flow is much decreased. Over 25 years ago studies of the percentage saturation of oxygen in the umbilical vein showed a dramatic fall after the 40th week of pregnancy. Although other workers at the time were unable to confirm these findings when using different methods of analysis, more recent studies have demonstrated striking histological changes in the placenta. The extreme vascularity of the chorionic villi regresses rapidly after full-term, when the capillaries become small and contracted. In an analysis of more than 5000 consecutive deliveries under personal supervision and conducted during the years 1953 to 1957 (before methods to measure fetal growth and assess placental function were available) I found prolonged pregnancy the most important single factor associated with asphyxia neonatorum, which could lead to perinatal mortality (Amiel, 1960)*.

REDUCING THE INCIDENCE OF POSTMATURITY
There can be little doubt, therefore, that the conditions discussed above − preterm delivery, intrauterine growth retardation and pro-

*Amiel, G. J. (1960). *J. Obstet. Gynaecol. Brit. Emp.*, **67**, 772.

longed pregnancy — all play a role in increasing perinatal mortality and morbidity. The incidence of these will be reduced by the following factors.

Ensuring a correct estimated date of delivery (EDD)
To achieve this it is important to take an accurate menstrual history and pay special regard to the causes for error (page 44). Uterine size on vaginal examination when performed by an experienced practitioner can usually be estimated to within 2 weeks in the first 14 weeks of pregnancy (usually, not invariably — see page 50). If the size of the uterus is as anticipated from the menstrual history, the EDD as calculated by Näegele's rule (page 43) may be considered satisfactory.

A positive pregnancy test if performed at an early stage and especially within 2 to 3 weeks after the first missed period is of value. Ultrasound measurements made in the first and second trimesters of pregnancy are useful aids, especially when marked discrepancies are found between the history as given by the patient and the size of the uterus. Fetal measurements made include crown—rump length, biparietal diameter and abdominal circumference, and experts in this field with modern equipment state that by measuring the first length (crown—rump) between the 7th and 12th week of pregnancy the gestational age may be determined to within 4 days. Serial ultrasound echograms are of special value in observing fetal intrauterine growth, particularly in the small-for-dates (SFD) baby.

Subjective symptoms experienced by the patient are of little use in estimating the duration of a pregnancy. The timing of fetal movements felt for the first time by the mother can be misleading. Multigravidae usually feel movements earlier than do primigravidae, and often long before the 18th week of pregnancy which is assumed to be the average time (see page 41). Fundal height gives only an approximate estimate of maturity. Radiography in late pregnancy to detect the fetal femoral and tibial epiphyses gives variable results but may indicate that the pregnancy has reached the last month.

Correcting conditions leading to fetal deprivation or preterm delivery
Measures to correct fetal deprivation include:

(1) Treatment of anaemias and nutritional deficiencies which are often associated with the socioeconomic status of the individual.
(2) The avoidance of smoking, especially to excess.
(3) The treatment of maternal disorders such as diabetes.
(4) The prevention of infection.
(5) The early recognition and treatment of pre-eclampsia and toxaemias.

(6) Stressing the importance of bedrest which improves the blood supply to the uterus and placenta, and admission to hospital when necessary.

Early diagnosis of multiple pregnancy and congenital anomalies

The administration of additional folic acid 1–5 mg daily may be of value in multiple pregnancies when the fetuses are liable to be dysmature. The value of this medication throughout pregnancy in all cases to prevent or reduce the incidence of fetal deprivation is not established.

Preventing preterm delivery as far as possible

This is aided by the most careful observation of all patients at special risk (as above), and ensuring that measures recommended and treatment given are adequate. Thus, for example, it is often advised that women with a twin pregnancy be admitted to hospital for a month between the 30th and 34th weeks so that adequate rest will reduce the incidence of pre-eclampsia and the need for early induction of labour. A *Shirodkar* suture around the internal os (page 151) may be of value in patients with a history of abortion or preterm deliveries believed to be due to an incompetent os. Hydramnios may improve with rest, and delivery of the fetus (if normal) may occasionally be delayed by withdrawing small amounts of liquor by abdominal amniocentesis.

Drugs used to suppress preterm labour in the third trimester have a limited value and include:

(1) Sedatives
(2) A group which acts upon the beta-receptor sites in the myometrium (see page 74) and by stimulating these inhibit uterine activity. They may be administered intravenously, intramuscularly or orally, and include:
   (a) Isoxsuprine, which being vasorelaxant is used primarily for its action on the beta-receptors in the walls of blood vessels and can cause prolonged hypotension. Thus it is preferable to consider the use of (b) or (c) below.
   (b) Salbutamol
   (c) Ritrodrine.
(3) Intravenous ethyl alcohol.
(4) Anti-inflammatory analgesic agents such as aspirin, indomethacin and naproxen are prostaglandin inhibitors and thus theoretically could be of value. Although trials with indomethacin suggest it is effective in suppressing labour, these agents can cross the placenta and possibly affect the fetus adversely, so as yet they are not to be recommended.

If preterm delivery appears likely, the administration of *cortico-steroids* to the mother for 2 or 3 days prior to delivery appears to accelerate fetal pulmonary maturity by enhancing the production of a lipoprotein called *surfactant*. This can reduce the incidence and severity of neonatal respiratory distress syndrome. Dosage varies, but betamethasone 4 mg intramuscularly every 8 hours or 12 mg daily for 2 days is often administered. Reports of maternal pulmonary oedema occurring in patients who have been given betamimetics and steroids make close observation essential when both drugs are used con-comitantly.

Monitoring placental efficiency

Tests for assessing placental function are numerous and include various hormone assays and enzyme estimations (such as heat-stable alkaline phosphatases). One of the best and most frequently used is the estimation of the amount of oestriol in a 24 hour collection of urine.

The fetal adrenals are responsible for the metabolism of most of the precursors of the oestrogens which then pass to the placenta and are converted to oestriol. Thus, both placenta and fetus must be active if the oestriol level is to be maintained. In pregnancy oestriol excretion is vastly increased, and this substance constitutes over 90% of the total amount of oestrogens in the urine. Thus, either oestriol or total oestrogen content may be calculated. A low level may be of sinister significance, and a falling level is even more important. Examinations may be made twice weekly and charted.

Measurement of plasma oestriol level may also be used and the results are obtainable more quickly. Human chorionic somatomammo-trophin (HCS — also known as human placental lactogen (HPL)), a hormone synthesized in the syncytial trophoblast, is also found in plasma. HCS radioimmunoassay in maternal blood is sometimes util-ized for assessment of placental function.

The tests, coupled with serial ultrasonography, are related to all the clinical features of the patient; maternal failure to gain weight may be significant.

Ensuring correct timing for induction of labour and delivery

This is of vital importance and tests to assist in the assessment of maturity and fetal wellbeing include numerous studies made on the amniotic fluid. The liquor of the forewaters may be studied transcer-vically with the aid of tapering conical amnioscopes. The volume may be judged and the presence or absence of meconium noted.

Other features studied on the liquor obtained by amniocentesis include the electrolyte content, acid—base equilibrium and creatinine concentration. The *cell content* can be studied by staining with Nile blue sulphate. Some cells shed into the amniotic fluid stain blue and others with no nucleus stain orange. The latter cells arise from fetal sebaceous glands and are not exfoliated until late pregnancy. The percentage of orange-staining cells increases as term is approached and generally if more than 10% are found to be 'orange-positive' the duration of pregnancy is 36 weeks or more. Not all observers, however, report a satisfactory correlation between orange-staining cells and gestational age.

Studies of the *lipid content* can provide the most useful information concerning the maturity of the fetal lungs. The presence of an adequate amount of the lipoprotein surfactant indicates that they are mature and this knowledge is of particular value where doubt exists about the necessity for immediate delivery. Maturity of the fetal lungs is shown by estimating the concentration of a phospholipid (lecithin), the level of which increases as term is approached. The *lecithin–sphingomyelin* (another phospholipid) or *LS ratio* is calculated. If this is high (over 2), the fetus and its respiratory centre may be considered to be mature and the danger of the infant developing hyaline membrane disease (or respiratory distress syndrome), the major risk of preterm delivery, is diminished.

Simple *'shake' tests* to estimate surfactant and fetal maturity have been described in which the amniotic fluid at various dilutions is shaken and examined for bubbles after 15 minutes. A positive result in dilutions of 1 in 4 or more is reassuring.

Monitoring the fetal condition during labour
The fetal heart rate may be continuously checked by ultrasonography recordings or by electrocardiography using a clip scalp electrode after the forewaters have ruptured. Changes in heart rate are related to uterine contractions which are recorded simultaneously. Furthermore, fetal blood sampling may be used to assess the fetal condition. The sample is obtained from the scalp and drawn into a special capillary tube. Fetal acidaemia indicates intrauterine hypoxia and the need to deliver the baby quickly.

The fetus *in utero* is better adapted to survive hypoxia than the neonate by virtue of its ability to utilize stored glycogen for anaerobic respiration. Anaerobic glycolysis leads to fetal acidosis with the accumulation of lactic and pyruvic acids. Growth-retarded fetuses have small livers, less subcutaneous fat, and muscle wasting is evident. Glycogen stores are thus deficient and these fetuses are unable to withstand any marked degree of hypoxia. Oxygen given to the mother in labour may be of some value although this has been questioned (see also Chapter 9).

Caring for the neonate by skilled staff
The care of the neonate by trained staff in a fully equipped neonatal care unit will diminish perinatal mortality. So patients in preterm labour, and especially if the gestation period is judged to be less than 34 weeks, should be given tocolytic agents if necessary and transferred before delivery to a centre with an intensive neonatal care unit; this is preferable to transporting the infant in an incubator. Even better is to identify all patients at high risk of preterm delivery so that satisfactory arrangements are made long before labour commences.

21

Induction of labour

The causes of spontaneous onset of labour are still obscure (see Chapter 7). Although a variety of factors is known to be involved in regulating uterine activity, hormonal influences almost certainly play a dominant role (page 74). Research continues and if definitive causes for initiating labour can be determined it may be possible to evolve a perfect medical method to induce it. The question will always arise as to the desirability and indications for induction of labour, its risks, its timing and the results to mother and baby.

Over the past 15 years the incidence of surgical induction of labour has almost trebled in many centres where the figure now approaches or even exceeds 30%. This increase is also associated with an increase in the percentage of hospital confinements compared with those taking place in the home. However, not all units report that this high rate

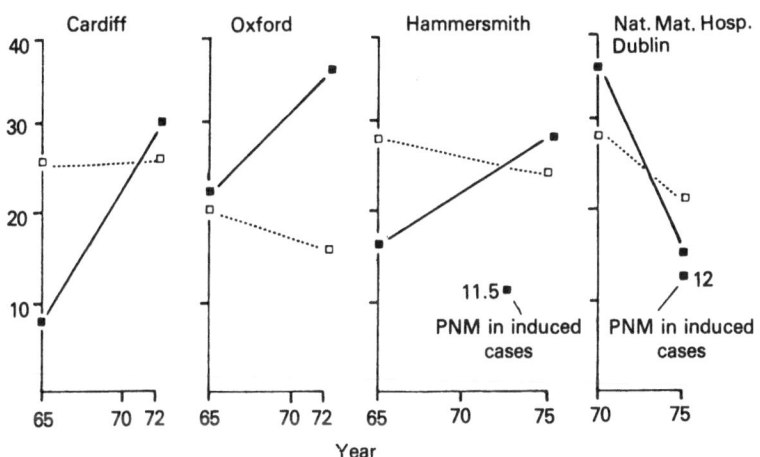

Figure 53 Induction rate and perinatal mortality rates from McClure Browne, J. C. and Dixon, G., *Browne's Antenatal Care*, Churchill Livingstone, Edinburgh, 1978, Eleventh Edition, with permission.

of surgical induction is associated with a fall in perinatal mortality (see Figure 53). The increased incidence of intervention in pregnancy and the active management of labour has received much public attention and most of the criticism appears to be adverse.

Yet the timely induction of labour, with current improved methods of achieving this, may be a major factor in reducing perinatal mortality, provided there are strong indications for induction. It has been stated with some truth that if there are grounds for surgical induction of labour, then there are grounds for performing caesarean section if induction fails to achieve delivery shortly after it has been performed. There can be little, if any, justification for inducing labour just for the convenience of members of the staff even though, with methods described below, delivery is usually achieved within 12 hours. It is to be sincerely hoped that the day will never come when a shortage of trained staff to give a 24 hour service every day of the year may make this a justifiable indication for induction!

However, I consider that labour can sometimes be initiated for the convenience and peace of mind of the mother. The psychological well-being of the patient is a factor often overlooked in discussions on this topic. It is important, when recommending induction, for the practitioner to discuss the matter fully with the patient, and her husband if possible, so that the indications are clearly appreciated. Of considerable importance in arriving at a decision will be factors such as the duration of pregnancy, the station of the presenting part (vertex or breech) and the condition of the cervix which is considered 'ripe' if at least partially effaced, soft, and 2 cm dilated (in other words, will admit a finger). If all conditions for induction are favourable and the pros and cons for the procedure are equally balanced, the views of the patient should be taken into account.

Indications for induction of labour

The main reasons include the following:

TOXAEMIAS OF PREGNANCY
See Chapter 14.

PROLONGED PREGNANCY
The problems associated with the correct assessment of the duration of pregnancy have been discussed earlier. It is in the post-term pregnancy that maternal peace of mind plays a large role in arriving at a decision concerning induction. Personal experience has shown that many women find the last days of pregnancy tedious, and if all conditions for induction are favourable, the pregnancy has progressed several days beyond the estimated date for delivery, and the patient so

desires, I arrange admission to hospital. If, however, the patient would prefer labour to commence spontaneously, and blood pressure and other findings including placental efficiency monitoring prove satisfactory, no intervention is necessary. Such patients with post-term pregnancies must be seen and assessed at least twice weekly.

DYSMATURITY

The timing of delivery of the small-for-dates baby will depend upon the answer to the question 'Will the baby fare better outside or inside the mother's uterus?' To a considerable extent the answer will depend upon the experience of the midwifery team and available facilities, the maternal condition and duration of pregnancy. The results of monit-oring placental function and fetal condition are vital aids to the obstetrician in arriving at the correct decision.

ACCIDENTAL AND UNAVOIDABLE APH

For treatment of accidental APH and first-degree placenta praevia see Chapter 17.

BREECH PRESENTATIONS

Personal preference is often to initiate labour about a week before term. I believe the fetal head post-term tends to become more ossified, so the sudden compression and decompression to which it is subjected in the rapid passage in and out of the maternal bony pelvis is assoc-iated with the slightly increased risk of cerebral haemorrhage. The breech with extended legs, or frank breech in which the buttocks are well applied to the cervix, is the most favourable podalic presentation.

PATIENTS WITH MINOR DEGREES OF DISPROPORTION

This category also includes *multiparae with a bad obstetric history*, such as difficult delivery of a large baby or unexpected intrauterine death near term or intrapartum. In these cases induction of labour at about 38 weeks should be considered. However, the statement on page ix is worthy of repetition, 'one of the essential features of the practice of obstetrics is the fact that there can be no hard and fast rules laid down to govern management. Each case is assessed individually and then reassessed at every subsequent antenatal examination before deciding upon the nature of the recommendations to be made to the patient.'

Other indications for induction of labour include fetal abnormal-ities, intrauterine death, rhesus isoimmunization, certain maternal dis-eases such as diabetes, and an unstable lie (especially where the fetal head tends to lie in the iliac fossa). This is corrected by external cephalic version and amniotomy is performed but the precautions must be taken as described on page 122.

Methods of induction

MEDICAL INDUCTION

Two methods, the OBE (oil, bath, enema) and bougies inserted into the uterus are mentioned for historical interest only. They belong in the past with other even more dangerous methods which included giving the patient quinine or oestrogens. Medical induction today consists of the administration of oxytocin and/or prostaglandin.

Oxytocin intravenous drip method

This method of induction has been in use for about 30 years and over this time there has been a tendency to increase the concentration of the solution used. This is not without risk as hypertonic incoordinate uterine action (see page 180) may result. Initially oxytocin was administered in so-called physiological dosage with 2 units of oxytocin in 1 litre of 5% glucose running at 15 drops per minute and continuing throughout labour. One regime found to be satisfactory is to set up a drip containing 5 units of oxytocin in 1 litre of 5% dextrose. The drip rate, electronically controlled, commences at 10 drops per minute and is increased ½-hourly by 10 drops per minute until satisfactory contractions (occurring every 3–5 minutes) are achieved and maintained. The flow is adjusted according to the nature of the contractions and never exceeds 60 drops per minute. If labour is not established by these means the regime is repeated, but the intravenous solution is made more concentrated by mixing 7.5 units or a maximum of 10 units of oxytocin in 1 litre of 5% dextrose.

Automatic infusion systems (such as the Cardiff pump) may be used, and this controls the infusion rate according to the strength and frequency of the contractions. This may well tend to diminish the total amounts of oxytocin and fluid administered and thereby prevent water intoxication. However, whatever drugs and devices are used, nursing and medical supervision remain essential throughout.

Oxytocin infusion is much more effective when combined with amniotomy or artificial rupture of the membranes (ARM). This is performed with the patient in the lithotomy position and full sterile and antiseptic techniques are used. The patient voids urine spontaneously prior to the procedure, and sedation, analgesia or anaesthesia are rarely necessary. The index finger is inserted through the cervix, the membranes are 'swept' and the forewaters ruptured with the aid of a Kocher's forceps. The hole in the membranes is then enlarged digitally. The Drew–Smythe catheter devised for rupturing the backwaters is now obsolete.

Prostaglandins

These may be given intravenously or orally, although vaginal pessaries and extra-amniotic administration via a urethral catheter inserted transcervically are also in use.

Prostaglandin E_2 (PGE_2) is now the substance of choice and for induction of labour ampoules containing 0.75 ml of a 1 mg/ml solution of dinoprostone in ethanol (one of the Prostin E_2 sterile solutions) are added to 500 ml of sterile normal saline or 5% dextrose. The bottle of the diluted solution contains 1.5 μg/ml, is labelled clearly and used with a drip set that delivers 60 drops per ml. The drip rate is started at 10 drops per minute, maintained for 30 minutes and if no uterine response is observed this rate is doubled. The rate is then increased by 10 drops per minute hourly, never exceeds 60 drops per minute (1.5 μg), and the lowest dose to produce satisfactory uterine response is maintained. Nausea, vomiting and diarrhoea, side-effects often reported with prostaglandin administration, are not common with this dosage regime, but there may be temporary local tissue irritation and venous erythema. The use of intravenous prostaglandin for induction is limited, as oxytocin is the substance of choice for the induction of labour.

Prostin E_2 tablets orally containing 0.5 mg dinoprostone may also be used. One tablet (and occasionally two tablets), given hourly up to 10 doses, is often effective in initiating labour, and this appears to be of value in ripening the cervix without initial amniotomy when early delivery is indicated. Alimentary system side-effects have not been troublesome and hypertonic uterine action has not occurred with this oral regime. Unlike oxytocin, PGE_2 does not have an antidiuretic effect, so it is of particular value in cases of severe toxaemia.

Advantages and disadvantages
Artificial rupture of the membranes followed immediately by oxytocin infusion usually effects delivery within 12 hours. Infusion, however, should not be routinely administered after artificial rupture of the membranes if the patient prefers to wait, but it is to be recommended about 12 hours later if labour is not established. The disadvantages of intravenous drip and monitoring fetal heart rate and uterine contractions, whereby a woman in labour is connected to various forms of equipment and may consider the process too mechanical and unnatural, must not be discounted. On the other hand, many women find interest and even pleasure in following progress with electronic aids and this is especially so if there has been full prior discussion with the patient.

Dangers of induction
The risks that may arise from induction of labour include the following.

FAILURE TO INITIATE LABOUR AND ACHIEVE DELIVERY

This may occur especially if the duration of pregnancy has been misjudged. 'Ripeness' of the cervix is only a single, albeit important, feature used in making a general assessment of the pregnancy. I have seen many multiparae with the cervix more than 2 cm dilated many weeks before the onset of labour, and in other cases an unripe cervix may be associated with postmaturity and placental insufficiency. Failure to initiate labour is more serious if artificial rupture of the membranes has been performed and risks to both mother and baby are increased.

INFECTION OF MOTHER AND BABY

Amniotitis, endometritis and intranatal fetal pneumonia may occur, especially after 24 hours of draining liquor. Thus, when this time has been reached, bacteriological examination of a vaginal swab is made and a broad-spectrum antibiotic is usually prescribed.

ANTEPARTUM HAEMORRHAGE

This may occur when artificial rupture of the membranes is performed in cases of hydramnios, but attempts to drain liquor slowly at first will minimize this risk. If necessary paracentesis abdominis may initially be performed to achieve this.

PROLAPSED CORD

The risk of this is slight if the head is engaged or entering the pelvis. The possibility of this complication is always kept in mind, and if the cord prolapses immediate caesarean section is indicated.

NEONATAL JAUNDICE

An increased incidence of hyperbilirubinaemia (bilirubin level 12 mg/100 ml or more) is reported where oxytocin infusion has been used with artificial rupture of the membranes.

Amniotic fluid embolism and uterine rupture (especially if unrecognized disproportion is present) are among the very rare but dangerous complications that could occur.

PERINATAL MORTALITY

Although most statistical surveys seen report a reduction in perinatal mortality associated with an increased incidence in induction rate this is not universal (see Figure 53). Induction of labour should, therefore, not be undertaken without positive indication.

22

The puerperium

The puerperium, usually accepted as the 6 weeks following delivery, is the time during which the genital organs should return to the normal non-pregnant state. The changes that occur are mostly of a retrogressive or involutionary nature. Vagina and vulva, pelvic floor and perineum recover from stretching and bruising while the most obvious of changes involve the uterus. Some puerperal bodily changes, however, are not those of involution as lactationary breast changes are progressive, a subject which is dealt with separately (Chapter 28).

The lying-in period is not a definitive number of days, but generally refers to the first 8 to 12 days postpartum. In the past the term referred to the time the normal patient remained in hospital. During this period the mother may experience difficulties with micturition or constipation and complain of discomfort in breasts or perineum. She may be concerned about varicose veins, abdominal striae or flabby abdominal wall musculature.

The physical and hormonal changes which are taking place so rapidly during the puerperium may in themselves contribute to the psychological state of the mother. She may be concerned about her general competence to deal with her new baby and this, together with domestic or financial problems, make it essential for all concerned with her care to ensure that the mother is comfortable, relaxed and confident. The management of labour and of the mother during the puerperium begins at her first prenatal examination and her psychological wellbeing is of paramount importance. With efficient and sympathetic care throughout, most mothers following an adequate rest after labour should feel well and be happy in their achievement.

The problems mentioned above are considered in this chapter, but first it is necessary to discuss the essentials of the physiological changes in the puerperium.

Physiological changes

THE UTERUS

After the completion of the third stage of labour, the fundus of the firmly retracted uterus will be palpable at, or just above, the level of the umbilicus. Daily abdominal palpation should show a progressive diminution in size, so that by the 10th day or shortly afterwards the organ is no longer palpable through the abdomen. Some practitioners measure the height of the fundus above the symphysis pubis and chart this graphically every day, while others estimate its height with the fingers. The important features, however, are to ensure that the estimation of size is made soon after the bladder has been emptied, that involution is progressive, the uterus not unduly tender, the patient remains apyrexial, and the lochia is normal.

The uterus immediately postpartum is reported to weigh approximately 1 kg, and in the non-pregnant state from 40 to 60 g. So complete involution of the uterus entails a reduction of weight by about 20 times in the 6 weeks postpartum. This is achieved largely by the action of proteolytic enzymes which cause degeneration of muscle fibres, and the soluble end-products of the breakdown being removed by the phagocytic action of polymorphs and macrophages in the bloodstream and lymphatics.

THE CERVIX

Immediately postpartum this is usually vascular and bruised and tends to hang down like a soft curtain, but within 24 hours it shortens and hardens. Although after 3 days the cervical canal will admit two fingers, within a month it is closed and normal on palpation.

LOCHIA

During the third stage of labour the placenta and membranes have separated through the deep spongy layer of the decidua. The blood vessels in the raw vascular area left inside the uterus thrombose and the site becomes covered with granulation tissue beneath which the endometrium starts to regenerate. Decidual debris, blood clot and shreds of fetal membranes lie superficially, all shed from the uterus after delivery as the *lochia*, and the discharge may continue for the entire puerperium or stop within a fortnight. For the first 3 days or so the lochia is red (lochia rubra) and consists mostly of blood from the placental site. But for the week or two that follow, the discharge darkens and thickens as blood diminishes, and increasing numbers of leucocytes appear with the degenerating decidual shreds and mucus from the cervix. This red-brown discharge (lochia serosa) becomes paler (lochia alba) and contains increasing numbers of bacteria, normally non-pathogenic, before it stops entirely.

The quantity, colour and odour of the lochia may all have a clinical significance. Excessive or prolonged blood loss, especially when accompanied by the passage of clots which is an abnormal occurrence, may be due to retained products of conception. This is more likely if involution of the uterus is inadequate and the placenta and/or membranes were found to be incomplete after delivery. It is, however, often normal for darkening lochia to become red again and increase slightly in quantity when physical activity is increased.

Although lochia has an odour which can vary from day to day and also with the individual patient, a frankly offensive smell suggests genital tract infection. Scanty amounts of lochia may be passed when uterine infection is present, but not when infection is associated with retained placental tissue. An obstruction caused by blockage or stenosis of the cervical canal may lead to the condition of *lochiometra* when no lochia whatsoever is passed but collects in utero. This condition is rarely seen, but if the obstruction is not relieved infection will result. Many obstetricians performing elective caesarean section in a primigravida with an 'unripe' cervix will pass a dilator through the cervical canal from the uterine cavity to avoid this condition.

DISORDERS OF MICTURITION

The disorders which may occur in the puerperium include retention of urine, dysuria and frequency, infection and incontinence.

Retention of urine

Retention can be due in part to dysuria following delivery and the causes include:

(1) Bruising and oedema around the urethra and base of the bladder.
(2) Psychological causes such as inability to pass water while lying in bed, using a bedpan or in the presence of other people in a ward. Early ambulation with assistance as required will generally obviate these causes.
(3) Spasm of the external urethral sphincter which may be associated with cause (2) above or perineal trauma or the presence of sutures.
(4) Failure of detrusor muscular activity following overdistension of the bladder during labour.

The overdistended bladder when there is retention of urine will cause the mother pain and distress and may often be avoided by the practitioner's knowledge of its causes. Reassurances given, adequate fluid intake, simple measures such as turning on a tap for the patient to hear the sound of running water and a warm bath as soon as possible may be curative. A patient after resting for 12 hours following delivery may generally have a shower to refresh her, even when her perineum contains sutures. It is important, however, to ensure that the surface on which she stands is not slippery and that she will not harm herself on any projections in the confined space of a shower cubicle. Catheterization of the bladder, a procedure to avoid whenever possible, is sometimes necessary and when this is so, the greatest care must be taken to avoid introducing infection.

Incontinence
This may be due to damaged fascial supports of the bladder in the urethrovesical area, or retention with overflow. True incontinence associated with fistulae may be either traumatic or due to ischaemic necrosis of bladder tissues following prolonged pressure. The former would be manifest immediately after delivery, and the latter 1 to 2 weeks later. Fortunately both are rare conditions in the United Kingdom.

Infection
For a fuller discussion see page 62 and Chapter 23.

THE BOWELS AND PERINEAL TEARS
Normal diet and early ambulation should result in no marked problems with bowel action during the lying-in period, but constipation for a few days after delivery is common. This is because there may be perineal and perianal discomfort, the abdominal wall musculature has been stretched and not regained its tone, and the bowel was emptied by enema at the onset of labour. If necessary a mild aperient such as senna (Senokot) may be given after 3 days.

Perineal tears are graded according to the extent of the damage. A *first-degree* tear involves the vaginal mucosa and skin of the perineum but almost invariably some fibres of the superficial perineal muscles are torn. A *second-degree* tear involves also the deeper layers of the perineal body while a *third-degree* tear extends into the anal sphincter and possibly the rectal mucosa. Good management of the second stage of labour (especially controlled delivery of the baby's head between contractions and taking particular care when the posterior shoulder is being eased out over the perineum) will prevent some tears. If there is any doubt whether or not an episiotomy is required it is better to perform it (page 102). Perineal tears do not necessarily indicate poor obstetrics as would the failure to repair 'small' tears (or so-called 'nicks') often associated with extensive muscular damage.

Bowel action is usually best left to nature, although in severe second-degree or third-degree tears a low residue diet is given. If the rectal mucosa has been sutured, some olive oil (approximately 130 ml) may be instilled into the rectum on the 5th day to facilitate the passage of a hard stool, but in second-degree tears this may be achieved by the oral administration of 10 or 15 ml of paraffin emulsion twice daily from the 3rd day onwards.

The tone of the musculature of the abdominal wall and of the pelvic floor will be improved by exercises (initially supervised by a physiotherapist). *Striae gravidarum* which form because of a breakdown of elasticity in the deeper layers of the skin of the abdominal wall, but can also be seen on breasts and thighs, may be associated with hormonal changes (? increased cortisol). Prenatal massage of the abdominal wall with olive oil or emollient creams may be of some value. The marks fade after many months but do not entirely disappear, and as much reassurance as possible will help the patient.

Psychological aspects
The importance of the psychological condition of the patient from the onset of pregnancy to after the puerperium has been stressed earlier, and disturbances can occur at any stage. The immediate days and weeks postpartum are of special importance. Physical discomfort, and involutionary and hormonal changes proceeding at a maximum rate, coupled with the mother's self-questioning about her competence to bring up her baby, all contribute to stress. The daily routine of life is considerably changed as sleep patterns are altered and marital relationships disturbed. Anaemia will increase maternal fatigue and this factor can and must be avoided. The baby's father, who should be involved as much as possible in the care of the patient during her pregnancy and labour, can often be a great help and support to his wife. The reaction of the parents to each other and to the baby should be observed and noted.

The '3rd day blues' in many patients who have undergone any major operation occurs as the emotional upset of the process of undergoing surgery becomes less intense. Similarly minor depression on about the 3rd day postpartum is no rarity. A confident cheerful and helpful attitude of all staff will usually overcome the transient 'blues' that may coincide with tenderness in the breasts as they fill with milk. Emotional lability in many mothers may be seen by their tearful reaction to a most simple question such as whether or not there has been any bowel action. Conflicting advice given to a mother by two different attendants concerning, for example, a baby-feeding problem which can be solved satisfactorily by two different methods, can be a shattering blow to her confidence, and should be avoided. Sedation is sometimes indicated for this transient depression, but generally a reassuring chat with a skilled and sympathetic attendant is preferable.

Even more support for both parents will be necessary if labour has resulted in the birth of an infant that failed to survive or was abnormal in any way. If the baby needs supervision in a special or intensive neonatal care unit, the mother should be kept fully informed and see her baby as often as possible.

A puerperal psychosis should be treated by a specialist psychiatrist with full team and facilities for therapy. The psychotic patient is confused, may hallucinate and temporarily lose the ability to coexist normally with her contacts. She may even be suicidal or harm her infant. Patients at special risk often have a previous history of psychological disorder or disturbed relationships both within and outside their family circle.

23

Puerperal pyrexia and infection

The puerperal woman with a pyrexia has an infection and for treatment to be effective it is necessary to investigate fully the nature, site and cause of the infection and whenever possible to identify the responsible agent and its source. 'Childbed fever' and the 'one-child sterility' due to bilateral tubal occlusion which ensued, fortunately are conditions of the past in most countries but infection still remains a hazard to both mother and the baby. Puerperal pyrexia used to be a notifiable disease in the United Kingdom and was then defined as a temperature of 100.4 °F (38 °C), or more occurring within 14 days of childbirth or miscarriage. Furthermore, the midwife's code of practice made it obligatory for a doctor to be informed if a patient's temperature was 99.4 °F (37.4 °C) or more on 3 successive days. Although puerperal pyrexia is no longer notifiable, the temperature levels quoted remain a most useful guide to alert the attendant to the possibility of significant infection.

Causes of puerperal pyrexia

These are:

(1) Infection of the genital tract
(2) Infection of the urinary tract (see pages 62 and 201)
(3) Breast complications
(4) Intercurrent infections such as upper respiratory tract infections, specific fevers, etc.

Genital tract infections

Puerperal pyrexia due to a genital tract infection is unlikely to be found within a few hours of the commencement of normal labour. It develops as a reaction to bacteria which have to gain access to the body via a *portal of entry*, and then multiply and elaborate their toxin, a process which usually takes a day or two to complete. The intact bag of membranes provides a barrier to ascending infection from the vagina and in normal labour the forewaters will not have ruptured until late in the first stage or at the beginning of the second stage. It is not uncommon to find a slight rise in temperature when recorded immediately postpartum and this finding is thus not usually due to genital tract infection. Labour itself, associated as it is with markedly increased muscular activity, is a mildly pyrexial process. But after the completion of labour, during which the placenta has separated through the deep spongy layer of the decidua basalis, the uterus is left with a large raw vascular area. This can provide as fruitful a zone for the growth of pathogenic organisms as a culture plate in an incubator. Knowledge of some facts of bacteriology will provide an invaluable aid to understanding the basic principles of the control of infection in obstetrics.

BACTERIA
These are classified and identified in the laboratory in various ways, and include:

(1) Morphological characteristics under the microscope such as

(a) cell shape; bacilli, for example, are rod-like and cocci are spherical or globular;
(b) arrangements of cells to each other: for example, streptococci are grouped in chains and staphylococci in clusters;
(c) presence or absence of motility, capsules and spores.

(2) Staining properties. The most commonly used diagnostic staining technique is Gram's stain. Bacteria that retain the methyl violet and iodine stain appear blue-black in colour and are referred to as Gram-positive, while those that do not but accept a red counterstain are Gram-negative.
(3) Biochemical and serological reactions, such as fermentation reactions.

Organisms which cause disease or pathology are *pathogens* whereas others are harmless *non-pathogens*. A *saprophyte* is a non-pathogen which obtains organic matter from dead tissue, while a *parasite* is an organism which obtains nourishment from another organism (the host). Not all parasites are harmful. Under certain conditions, such as anaemia and the presence of haemorrhagic, bruised or lacerated tissues, non-pathogenic organisms may become pathogenic. *Aerobic* organisms flourish in the presence of free oxygen, whereas *anaerobes* live in the absence of free oxygen or air.

Some examples of bacteria which may be of importance in puerperal infection are given below.

Staphylococci
These may be present on the normal skin or in the nose while other strains (*Staphylococcus pyogenes*) are pathogenic and cause infections and frankly purulent lesions such as boils and breast abscesses. Many strains of the ubiquitous staphylococcus exist and may be identified by techniques known as *phage typing*. Hospital strains of staphylococcus can become resistant to many antibiotics and thus be dangerous.

Haemolytic streptococci
These exist in many groups and subgroups with many of the pathogens often in group A. Streptococcal infections include sore throats, tonsillitis, scarlet fever, erysipelas, and may also be associated with rheumatic fever and acute nephritis. This organism used to be a major cause of puerperal sepsis but antibiotics diminished its importance and its serious role. Also the organism appeared to lose much of its virulence some decades ago.

Anaerobic streptococci
These are found in mucous membranes and skin of normal healthy people. They may be found in over 30% of normal vaginae.

Escherichia coli (E. coli)
These are part of the normal flora of the intestinal tract and a common cause of urinary tract infection. Another of this family of enterobacteria is *Bacillus proteus* which is present in faeces and may also infect the urinary tract.

Countless other organisms may cause puerperal infection of the genital tract, and the organisms and their sensitivity are determined by the bacteriologist. The anaerobic organism of gas gangrene, the *Clostridium welchii*, may be cultured from a vaginal or wound swab and be of no significance in the total absence of clinical evidence of this serious infection. The importance of the causative agent in puerperal infections changes with time, place and the facilities available.

SOURCE OF INFECTION
Infection may be acquired in three ways as follows:

(1) *Exogenous*, in which the infection arises from an outside source.
(2) *Endogenous*, whereby an organism already present in the area becomes pathogenic. The anaerobic streptococcus provides an

example of this. Present in a healthy vagina it may become a pathogen when haemorrhagic tissues have been inadequately repaired, and especially when the patient is anaemic or debilitated. (3) *Autogenous*, in which the infecting organism comes from another part of the patient herself. *Escherichia coli* may be an example of this when the coliform organism came from the patient's own gut.

Infections acquired by methods (1) and (3) may be spread by touch or droplets which arise from the nose, throat or respiratory tract of attendant, relative, or the patient herself (autogenous). Droplets which issue from the mouth in two main streams as shown in Figure 54 may infect wounds, clothes, skin, instruments, gloves and gowns. Dust, too, is infected and is the most important *intermediate carrier* of infection.

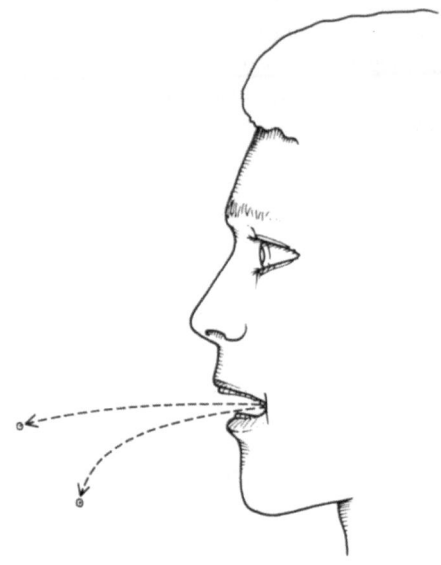

Figure 54 Droplet infection

PORTALS OF ENTRY

The *portals of entry* of bacteria in genital tract infection, in order of importance, are:

(1) The placental site
(2) The lacerated cervix
(3) The lacerated vagina
(4) The lacerated perineum and vulva.

Infection may remain localized, as perhaps when the portal of entry is (4) above and a sutured perineum does not heal properly, or spread causing cellulitis, peritonitis, thrombophlebitis or generalized septicaemia.

PREVENTION AND CONTROL OF GENITAL TRACT INFECTION
Factors which determine whether infection spreads or not include:

(1) The magnitude of the infection; for example, a normal throat may contain haemolytic streptococci, but a sore throat may teem with virulent streptococci.
(2) The virulence of the organism.
(3) The local conditions, for instance whether lacerated tissues are present.
(4) The general defences of the patient: hence anaemia must be avoided.
(5) Treatment given.

In hospitals in the United Kingdom the prevention and control of infection is usually exercised under the guidance of a specialized team headed by a bacteriologist. All trained personnel in a maternity service, however, must be aware of the essential features involved, and this means knowledge of the bacteria, their source, mode of spread and portals of entry to the genital tract. The basic principles of prevention and control of genital tract infection in obstetrics are as follows:

(1) Keep the patient away from any possible source of infection. Thus staff, relatives and visitors even with minor infections such as coryza or paronychia should be excluded from the labour and lying-in wards and from contact with the mother and her neonate when possible.
(2) Sterility for all deliveries and operative procedures must be of the highest order available. Disposable items such as syringes sterilized by gamma-radiation are excellent, and hospitals may be served by a central sterilizing depot (CSD). The ideal antiseptic will eliminate bacteria without damage to tissues, skin or mucosa of the patient and baby, and solutions and creams containing chlorhexidine and emulsions with hexachlorophane are of value. Masks are not used so frequently today, although a sound mask properly worn provides an effective barrier to the passage of, for instance, a haemolytic streptococcus. In the past, masks were worn by attendants when the patient's breasts or vulva were exposed and by all personnel entering a nursery. This is no longer customary or necessary practice and the healthy

neonate is best nursed in a cot by the mother's bedside. Certainly a defective mask or one improperly used always constituted a greater hazard than no mask at all. If a mother is breastfeeding and has even a minor throat infection she should, however, be given a mask to wear while feeding her infant.

(3)   As dust is an important intermediate carrier of infection, floors should not be swept but wet-mopped or vacuum-cleaned. This should not be done, nor bedding disturbed, immediately prior to infant feeding or exposure of the perineum for any purpose. Fabrics for bedding and curtains, decor including light fixtures and such, must be selected with care and a balance struck between aesthetic acceptability and dust-holding capability! Crevices and cracks in floors and walls should not be permitted.

(4)   Overcrowding considerably increases the risk of cross-infection and consideration of bed spacing in a ward is important. The provision of showers and bidets is an advantage.

(5)   Patients with infections should be isolated, examined fully, and bacteriological investigation should be conducted to identify the responsible organisms and their sensitivity. Treatment must be given at the earliest opportunity and in adequate dosage and will usually continue for a minimum of 48 hours after clinical signs of the infections have disappeared

(6)   In some units, staff and all patients on entry have nose and throat swabs investigated routinely. If a patient shows any clinical evidence of genital tract infection a vaginal swab, too, should be taken and investigated.

24

Thromboembolism

Varicose veins

Varicose veins in the legs are common in pregnancy, especially in multigravidae, and on the whole are best treated conservatively, although injection with sclerosant agents (such as sodium tetradecyl sulphate – STD injection) is occasionally performed. Varicosities may appear in the early weeks of pregnancy when blood vessels become more distensible owing to the increase in blood volume and loss of tone of the involuntary muscle in the vessel walls. This is part of the generalized hypotonia of unstriped muscle associated with the altered hormone status of pregnancy. Increased amounts of circulating progesterone are cited as the main causal factor for varicose veins, haemorrhoids, and also for pyelitis (hypotonic ureteric muscle), heartburn (cardiac sphincter), and constipation (bowel wall). Later in pregnancy varicose veins become more pronounced as venous flow is obstructed by pressure from the enlarging uterus. Treatment is to recommend that the patient rest with feet elevated as much as possible, and support with thigh-length elastic net stockings, or elasticated surgical tubular stockinette is often useful. Stockings or stockinette should be put on each morning before rising.

Varicosities also appear on the vulva and less commonly in the vagina. Vulval varicosities are sometimes very prominent and attempts to provide support with firmly applied pads are not very effective. Sclerosing injections are used but as much bedrest as possible is advisable. Haemorrhage from veins does occur but is rare, and a patient concerned about this possibility should be informed that rest and digital pressure on the bleeding point will suffice to stem the bleeding until expert advice is available.

The essentials of blood clotting are mentioned on page 160. In pregnancy there is an increased tendency to thrombosis because of the physiological blood changes that occur, including an increase in fibrinogen, prothrombin and number of platelets which also become more adhesive. Physical inactivity, excessive bedrest, anaemia and infection

211

especially in the presence of damaged tissues all add to the risk of thrombosis and are factors more commonly encountered in the puerperium. A further hazard would be the administration of oestrogens which increase blood coagulability, so the use of this hormone is contraindicated at all stages of pregnancy and the puerperium. The widespread use of the hormone to inhibit lactation was shown to increase the risk of pulmonary embolism. At special risk are grandmultiparae over 35 years of age, adipose women, patients with a previous history of thrombotic episodes, and those delivered by caesarean section. Some races in Africa and the Far East appear to have an immunity from deep vein thrombosis.

Superficial thrombophlebitis
Tenderness and erythema over an indurated vein, usually in the calf or thigh, indicates superficial thrombophlebitis. The condition by itself does not constitute any marked risk and is best treated by active leg movements with the patient wearing a support stocking. If tenderness is marked and it is too painful for the patient to be ambulant, active leg movements while in bed are encouraged and a bed cradle to remove the pressure of the bed covers is of value. Local dressings used to give relief include glycerine and ichthyol applications and kaolin poultices. Phenylbutazone orally for a few days may give relief, but must not be used with coumarin-type anticoagulants, and should be stopped if there are any side-effects (gastrointestinal irritation, rashes or oedema). It may be used with discretion in the puerperium.

Deep vein thrombosis
This can develop at any stage during a pregnancy although for reasons stated above the condition occurs more commonly during the puerperium. The complication of pulmonary embolus is today the most important cause of maternal mortality in England and Wales, though the number of deaths from this condition has diminished progressively over the past 20 years, particularly when following vaginal delivery (incidence is currently about 1 in 100 000). Factors contributing to this diminution are early ambulation and the avoidance of anaemia, traumatic delivery and infection. The decline in maternal deaths from pulmonary embolus in the antepartum period or following caesarean section has, however, been far less dramatic.

The incidence of deep vein thrombosis in Europeans is in the region of 0.2 to 0.3% and the diagnosis is sometimes difficult to make on clinical grounds. It must always be considered when a patient complains of pain or discomfort in the legs – usually the earliest symptom of the condition. Deep thrombosis is most commonly found in the calf veins, and there is tenderness over the affected area. The calf muscles are relaxed and palpation is best performed by requesting the recumbent patient to flex her knees to approximately a right angle and rest the soles of her feet flat on the couch or bed. Oedema may be marked, although the very swollen 'white leg' (phlegmasia alba dolens) caused by ileofemoral thrombosis in the prenatal period is rarely seen today. *Homan's sign*, or pain produced in the calf by dorsiflexion in the foot, is often positive.

Some authorities distinguish thrombophlebitis in which the infective or inflammatory element is marked, from phlebothrombosis which can occur in a deep calf vein with little or no inflammatory reaction. Whether this differentiation is valid is correctly questioned by many and, indeed, if there are two varieties of thrombosis, the one with a largely infective element is less likely to form emboli as the clot becomes firmly attached to the wall of the blood vessel. The 'silent' phlebothrombosis with fewer warning symptoms is more dangerous.

DIAGNOSIS

Aids to the diagnosis of deep vein thrombosis include:

(1) Ultrasonic examination using the Doppler effect to study blood flow sounds in the femoral vein, with a small portable ultrasonic machine.

(2) Venography. A radio-opaque medium injected into the veins of the foot may show a filling defect.

(3) Thermography. An affected leg is warmer than normal.

(4) Radioactive isotope injection with labelled fibrinogen; [^{125}I]fibrinogen is recommended but rarely used, and reports indicate that radioactive iodine may be present in milk and lochia following this test.

TREATMENT

Deep vein thrombosis in pregnancy is treated with the anticoagulant heparin which increases the blood-clotting time by inhibiting the action of thrombin and other coagulation factors (such as factor X). Intravenous injection achieves this action almost immediately and its effect lasts up to 6 hours. Symptoms are rapidly relieved with relative safety and the heparin effect of haemorrhage can be reversed if necessary by an intravenous injection of 1% protamine sulphate solution. Dosage is controlled by repeated studies of blood coagulation time and an average dose may be in the order of 10 000 units every 4–6 hours. Continuous intravenous administration of heparin in saline or glucose requires the most careful monitoring and also tends to curb the patient's active movements. Active leg exercises while in bed and ambulation as early as possible are important, and the symptom of pain is usually the only restricting factor. Pain in the leg disappears quickly after the commencement of treatment, and oedema subsides. A daily measurement of the girth of the thigh and calf of both legs should be recorded as a guide to the amount of swelling present and the rate of its subsidence.

Heparin therapy is continued for at least 7 days by which time the patient should be fully ambulant and treatment is tailed off gradually. Some patients, particularly those with a previous history of thrombo-embolism may require anticoagulation throughout the pregnancy and puerperium. Long-term therapy is best achieved with low dosage sub-cutaneous heparin which may be self-administered twice daily while heparin levels are estimated weekly. This therapy is temporarily suspended or reduced at the onset of labour to avoid haemorrhage. Epidural anaesthesia is best avoided in these patients as the risk of local bleeding is increased.

Oral anticoagulation with a drug such as warfarin should not be used in pregnancy or labour, as it has a more prolonged action which is less readily reversed (by vitamin K_1), and unlike heparin it crosses the placenta. In addition to the hazard of haemorrhagic accidents to the fetus, teratogenic effects have also been reported. The dangers of oral anticoagulation in pregnancy are reduced if it is used in the mid-trimester, and administration in late pregnancy should be stopped several weeks before delivery. Warfarin, therefore, is thus best avoided in pregnancy. It is also excreted in breast milk and so its use in the puerperium should be restricted to mothers who are not breastfeeding their babies.

Pulmonary embolism
Pulmonary embolus, if it occurs, requires a higher initial dose of intravenous heparin, and in addition to oxygen other drugs such as morphine and digoxin are used. The use of thrombolytic agents such as streptokinase or surgical therapy (embolectomy, or even more rarely, inferior vena caval ligation) would be decided by the appropriate experts and, indeed, all anticoagulant therapy should be conducted under the supervision of a consultant haematologist.

Prophylaxis of thromboembolism in patients at special risk, such as those undergoing caesarean section, may be achieved by giving the patient an infusion of 1 litre of Dextran 70 at the time of delivery. Apparently the solution makes a thrombus more susceptible to natural fibrinolysis and the infusion may be commenced after induction of the anaesthesia for caesarean section. Dextran 70 should not be given to a patient receiving heparin as the risk of haemorrhage would be increased, and the infusion should cease immediately if there is any suspicion of anaphylactoid reaction. The latter is a rare occurrence, more commonly seen in patients with a history of asthma.

25

Heart disease, pulmonary tuberculosis and venereal diseases in pregnancy

Heart disease

Although both the incidence (now below 1% of all cases) and nature of heart disease in pregnancy has altered over the past 30 years, the condition remains one of considerable importance and is a major cause of maternal death in most countries of the western world. Rheumatic heart disease which accounted for over 90% of all cases seen before 1950 has declined in both incidence and severity in both the United Kingdom and the United States, and now congenital heart lesions account for approximately 30% of the total. The reasons for these changes include:

(1)   The discovery and use of antibiotics in the early 1940s; penicillin played a major role in reducing and controlling the incidence of streptococcal infections which precede rheumatic fever.
(2)   The improved social conditions which diminish the spread of infection.
(3)   The survival of more patients with congenital heart disease, many of whom have been cured by surgery and have become pregnant.

Hypertension and coronary artery disease, although common causes of cardiopathy in later life, are infrequently factors in pregnancy. Other rare causes of heart disease found in pregnancy are hyperthyroidism, anaemia and syphilis.
Cardiac diseases are important as increased demands are made on the heart in pregnancy for the following reasons:

(1)   Altered haemodynamics of pregnancy. The increase in total blood volume which commences towards the 12th week of pregnancy has been discussed earlier (see physiological hydraemia, page 56). The increase in plasma volume may be as high as 50% in the last trimester, and the heart works harder to keep the fluid circulating. There

is an associated increase in cardiac output which is achieved largely by an increase in stroke volume, although the heart rate also tends to increase slightly as the pregnancy nears term. Much of the increased blood flow is directed via the hypertrophied uterine arteries, and this is important as an adequate supply to the placental area is essential for fetal wellbeing.

(2) The patient's weight increases in pregnancy so all physical activity involves the expenditure of additional energy.

(3) Reduced oxygenation of blood. The enlarged uterus may slightly reduce the respiratory movements of the diaphragm by displacing it upwards. This was thought possibly to reduce oxygenation of the blood at a time when increased oxygenation was desirable. However, when pregnant a woman breathes with greater expansion of the chest wall and also more rapidly (? hormone effect), and impairment of diaphragmmatic movement plays little or no part in increasing the demands on cardiac function.

DIAGNOSIS
The altered haemodynamics and increased blood flow through the large vessels found in every pregnancy are responsible for the very common finding of a heart murmur on routine auscultation. A systolic ejection murmur, generally soft and short in duration, may be audible over the base of the heart at some stage in pregnancy in the majority of patients. As with all associated diseases of pregnancy, the obstetrician and the appropriate specialist colleague collaborate in the care of the patient who has organic heart disease. However, it is also important to ensure that a patient is not worried unduly by referral to a cardiological department because she has the physiological or 'haemic' murmur of pregnancy just described. Previous medical history, obstetric history if any, personal history (for instance, did the patient have a normal school life with no restrictions on physical activity?) and present exercise tolerance (such as, is the patient able to climb stairs and perform domestic or other tasks with no undue dyspnoea, cyanosis or palpitations?) are all of significance in aiding the assessment of cases. Then, if there is doubt concerning cardiac findings, it is preferable to seek cardiological opinion, giving the patient as much reassurance as possible (for instance by stating that pregnancy murmurs are a very common finding and seeking a further opinion is the usual routine).

PRINCIPLES OF MANAGEMENT
Delivery of the baby of a mother with heart disease should occur when the patient is in the best possible condition that rest and therapy can achieve (assuming that the fetus is not in imminent danger, when the

most careful reappraisal of all factors is essential). This, and the avoidance of maternal cardiac failure are the aims of prenatal supervision. The latter should involve more frequent visits than usual, and in the first two trimesters a prenatal consultation at least fortnightly is desirable. The arrangements for examinations must take into account the patient's social conditions and steps taken to ensure that she does not have to make excessively tiring journeys. Specialists, general practitioners, midwives and social workers may all participate in patient care.

The nature of the cardiac disease and the functional capacity of the heart (in other words, the exercise tolerance of the patient), are both important considerations. Functional grading of cases as recommended by the New York Heart Association in 1939 may be summarized as follows:

Grade 1   No limitation of physical activity – evidence of cardiac disease is apparent only on examination with stethoscope, electrocardiogram etc.

Grade 2   Slight limitation of activity – dyspnoea on hurrying or heavy work, but able to walk leisurely on flat surface, or climb stairs slowly.

Grade 3   Marked limitation of activity – slight exertion causes dyspnoea, and other symptoms manifest include cyanosis, palpitations and oedema.

Grade 4   Dyspnoea at rest – the patient would normally be in hospital in cardiac failure; breathlessness while propped up in bed (orthopnoea) is present with other symptoms as above; pulsation may be seen in the neck veins and liver may be enlarged.

This classification is still widely used although condemned by some authorities because it may be difficult to apply and with certain lesions heart failure can develop suddenly. Thus, for example, a patient with rheumatic mitral stenosis and a heart of normal size can develop failure and acute pulmonary oedema with little warning. This occurs as the plasma volume expands and produces an increased flow through a small valve opening of fixed diameter. The sudden pressure rise in the left atrium behind the tight valve is transmitted back to the pulmonary vasculature causing pulmonary oedema. These patients may benefit by valvotomy which is much better performed before embarking on pregnancy. However, operation during pregnancy may be required since if failure develops antepartum it may recur during delivery. Such surgery in the gravid patient does carry some added risk.

Congestive cardiac failure (failure of output from both right and left ventricles) is also encountered in pregnancy. It usually develops more slowly than the acute left ventricular failure seen with pure mitral stenosis. It is associated with mixed valve lesions and often myocardial damage. Medical management rather than surgery is usually more appropriate.

Patients with *congenital heart lesions* on the whole do well in pregnancy and in labour, especially if cyanosis is not a feature of the disease. However, the specific lesion is important. Many cases will have had a surgical repair before pregnancy. A *patent ductus arteriosus* with its loud 'machinery' murmur will usually have been ligated or divided before puberty, but if necessary surgical treatment during pregnancy can be undertaken. The narrow portion of the artery in the condition of *coarctation of the aorta* can also be resected in pregnancy to avoid rupturing. The condition is recognized by the association of hypertension and a delayed femoral pulse. *Eisenmenger's syndrome* (pulmonary hypertension with congenital anomalies of the heart) is associated with a high maternal and perinatal mortality rate, and although many cases are delivered, pregnancy is better avoided. All these conditions are best managed by specialized teams.

The aim of management is, as stated above, to ensure that the patient is kept in the best possible condition. Adequate rest is most important and a mid-afternoon rest with the feet raised for an hour or two should be recommended as routine throughout pregnancy. Social conditions, care of other children in the family, their age and whether or not they are at school during the day may be important, as is the availability of help from friends or family. Hospitalization should be readily available, especially in the last trimester. The added hazard of pre-eclampsia developing is less likely with adequate rest.

Factors which can precipitate failure and must be avoided include anaemia, insomnia (sedation may be indicated) and infection. Crowded areas when colds and upper respiratory tract infections are prevalent are best avoided and if the patient develops an infection antibiotic cover should be freely given. When bacteria may be released into the bloodstream, such as at dental extractions and during delivery even in normal labour, a broad-spectrum antibiotic should be prescribed to patients with valve lesions. This will ensure in almost all cases that the bacteraemia will not lead to bacterial endocarditis.

TREATMENT
Drug therapy
Digoxin, or other cardiac glycosides, are not always indicated for patients with heart disease in pregnancy but may be used if necessary. Digitalization would certainly be required if atrial fibrillation were present or threatening (such as multiple ectopic beats). Diuretic

therapy with frusemide, for example, relieves failure although it is preferably avoided in the first 4 months of pregnancy. Potassium supplements should be given with diuretics if the latter are to be taken for some weeks.

If a patient with valve lesion develops atrial fibrillation during a pregnancy there is an increased danger of thromboembolism and it may be necessary to consider anticoagulant therapy. Women with prosthetic heart valves are probably taking this therapy prophylactically and a pregnancy is better avoided. If anticoagulation is to be used, heparin should be administered as discussed under thromboembolism (Chapter 24).

Surgery
This was discussed briefly above, page 219.

MANAGEMENT IN LATE PREGNANCY AND LABOUR
Monitoring of placental efficiency should be commenced at about the 32nd week of pregnancy, and delivery avoided if possible while a patient is in functional grade 3 or 4. If there is no pressing obstetrical reason for urgent delivery near term, and obstetrician and cardiologist consider further therapy will improve the patient's general condition, the therapy must continue. All patients may benefit by rest in hospital for several days before labour. Surgical induction of labour is on the whole better avoided as the risk of infection is increased, but if the procedure is necessary, there should be broad-spectrum antibiotic cover.

In the first stage of labour the patient must be kept comfortable in a 'propped-up' position and oxygen may be administered if there is dyspnoea; epidural analgesia is also of value (see page 100). The second stage of labour is often rapid and easy and this may be due to the soft parts and especially the pelvic floor being easily stretched owing to the accompanying pelvic congestion. If, however, advance in the second stage is not rapid, and particularly if the patient's pulse rate is rising, assistance with forceps and/or episiotomy is given. The third stage of labour is managed normally.

Antibiotic cover for labour and the 5–7 days postpartum is given to all cases as described above. Although as much rest as possible during the lying-in period is indicated, active leg movements are encouraged and early ambulation is preferable to avoid thromboembolism.

Although the spontaneous onset of labour and vaginal delivery are ideal, occasionally caesarean section may be indicated for obstetric reasons (such as disproportion, or increasingly severe pre-eclampsia). Termination of pregnancy because of heart disease is rarely necessary.

Postnatally the patient will require reassessment and advice from the cardiologist, and family planning advice should be offered (see Chapter 27).

Pulmonary tuberculosis

In the United Kingdom 40 years ago the incidence of active pulmonary tuberculosis in apparently healthy young adults was in the region of 0.5%, but the figure began to fall dramatically in the 1950s so that within a decade cases in pregnancy were rarely seen. Thus, in view of radiation hazards to the fetus, routine chest X-ray in early pregnancy as practised in most centres was abandoned. However, the incidence of tuberculosis in the United Kingdom is now increasing again, being higher in women from Pakistan and India, in those living under poor social conditions and in those with a family history or history of contact with the disease. Although pregnancy and labour have no adverse effects on the disease process, early diagnosis is important because the neonate has no immunity and must not be exposed to active tubercle bacilli. Furthermore the care of a baby will involve additional maternal stress and strain. Thus a patient at high risk of the disease or in whom there is clinical evidence of chest infection should have a chest X-ray. The possible teratogenic effects of radiation are most marked in the second month of gestation and the optimum time for X-ray is in the 14th to 16th week. One large film is taken and the radiographer should be made aware of the pregnancy so that abdomen and pelvis are protected. Miniature films used in population-screening programmes are contraindicated as radiation is not so well localized. Single chest X-rays may be taken earlier than the 14th week if there is concern on clinical grounds, as radiation hazards (leukaemia, bone cancer, genetic mutation and congenital abnormalities) are very small. All cases of suspected tuberculous infection should have sputum or laryngeal swabs examined for bacilli.

Treatment for the pregnant woman will be on the advice of the chest physician but some essentials of the disease are discussed below.

ACTIVE DISEASE

Full antituberculous therapy regimes are usually prescribed and drugs commonly used include streptomycin, para-aminosalicylic acid (PAS) and isonicotinic acid hydrazide (isoniazid or INH). Prolonged use of streptomycin can damage the vestibular division of the auditory (8th cranial) nerve and produce ataxia, vertigo and deafness. The drug can cross the placenta and cause congenital deafness although the level of streptomycin in fetal blood at birth is much less than that found in the mother. Parents, however, should be informed of this small risk and hearing tests performed on the infant at an early opportunity.

OBSTETRIC MANAGEMENT

Many of the features discussed in the management of patients with heart disease are also applicable to tuberculosis. Anaemia, added infections such as coryza or other upper respiratory tract infections, and insomnia are to be avoided. Adequate rest is advisable but hospitalization is usually unnecessary unless active open disease is present or the patient is toxic or pyrexial. Chemotherapy has reduced the need for surgical treatment which is usually best deferred, and although the maintenance of an artificial pneumothorax or pneumoperitoneum is possible it is not often performed. A pneumoperitoneum however, must not be renewed in the second half of pregnancy.

Assistance for delivery in the second stage of labour should be given if progress is not rapid and achieved with ease, and epidural analgesia is of value here. The third stage of labour is managed normally.

It is of interest to note that although careful microscopic examination of the placenta may often reveal the presence of the lesions of the disease (tubercles) congenital tuberculosis is very rare. The risk to the baby lies in the fact that it has no natural immunity to the disease yet may be in close contact with the infection, especially if any member of the household has open tuberculosis. The newborn are thus protected by being vaccinated with *BCG* (*bacille Calmette-Guérin*) generally in the first week of life.

BCG and Mantoux test

BCG is a bovine strain of tubercle bacilli which has been treated so that the organisms lose the ability to produce the disease (pathogenicity) but maintain the antigenic property (the property to stimulate the formation of antibodies). It takes approximately 6 weeks for the baby to form the antibodies to develop immunity and when this has been achieved the baby's tuberculin (Mantoux) test should be positive. If the test gives a negative result, repetition 2 weeks later is indicated. In the 6-week period during which immunity is developing, the baby must not be exposed to possible infection, and is segregated from its mother only if she has open disease. If this applies, segregation is maintained until the infant's Mantoux test becomes positive.

Breastfeeding may be allowed if the disease is quiescent and was inactive before pregnancy occurred. The chest physician should see the patient 1 month after delivery when a chest X-ray is usually arranged and further management discussed.

Venereal diseases

By definition, venereal infections (the term is derived from Venus, the Roman goddess of love) are those acquired or transmitted by sexual intercourse. By statute in England and Wales, venereal *diseases* comprise only gonorrhoea, syphilis and chancroid or soft sore – the latter seen in women only rarely. Several other infections, however, can be acquired venereally and these include trichomonal and candidal vaginitis, herpes genitalis, viral warts or condylomata acuminata, lymphogranuloma venereum and granuloma inguinale.

The two venereal diseases most often seen in the United Kingdom are gonorrhoea and syphilis, and it is most important that the infections are recognized, identified and treated so that the infant remains unaffected. These conditions and vaginitis associated with trichomonas and candida which are not uncommon in pregnancy are discussed below.

GONORRHOEA

Gonorrhoea is due to infection with the gonococcus, an intracellular Gram-negative diplococcus (that is, found in pairs). The incubation period of the disease is usually from 2–10 days, but may be as long as 16 days. Although typically the infection causes:

(1) cervicitis which is associated with a purulent discharge,
(2) urethritis with frequency of micturition, dysuria and discharge, and
(3) Bartholinitis,

the presence of the organism may well be missed on a direct smear and is frequently masked by a concomitant trichomonas infection. Discharge from cervix or urethra (after massaging the latter through the anterior vaginal wall) is best examined by direct transfer with a sterile platinum loop to plates containing a special culture medium. Examination of a high vaginal swab is of little value and complement fixation tests on serum so often performed in the past are unreliable. These are factors which stress the point that the diagnosis and treatment of suspected gonorrhoea is best left to a venereologist working in a specialized centre where, too, it would be easier to arrange investigation of contacts who may be affected.

The infection is now a very common one. In the early 1940s the incidence of gonorrhoea in the United Kingdom rose due to the social disruption caused by war. In England and Wales nearly 50 000 new cases were treated in 1946. Penicillin played an important part in the progressive decline in numbers of new cases in the following decade, but unfortunately this trend was not maintained and the disease is far more common today than in the 1940s. Oral contraceptives and increased sexual permissiveness are doubtless responsible for the increase, but the gonococcus itself has developed resistance to penicillin so that higher dosage becomes necessary when treating the condition.

The purulent vaginal and urethral discharge has been mentioned above, but signs and symptoms of the disease in the female are often minimal or absent. Arthritis and iritis are among the rare complications that can follow untreated or inadequately treated gonorrhoea, but salpingitis causing bilateral tubal blockage is common. There is an additional hazard associated with pregnancy in that though the disease has been quiescent for some years, the infant's eyes may become infected by organisms which have persisted in the cervical glands or paraurethral ducts (page 13) and which have been expressed during parturition. A purulent discharge from a baby's eyes is called *ophthalmia neonatorum* and if gonococcal in origin, blindness can result if proper treatment is not instituted immediately. Bacteriological examination of the discharge is conducted and penicillin eye drops (10 000 units per ml) instilled hourly initially, in addition to systemic administration of penicillin.

Treatment
Treatment regimes for gonorrhoea may differ slightly but might consist of:

(1)   Procaine penicillin − one injection of 2.4 mega-units which used to be recommended is associated with a small failure rate, and this dose is now mostly doubled.
(2)   Probenecid − 1 g orally prior to penicillin will prolong the action of the latter.
(3)   Oral ampicillin − on average 500 mg 6 hourly for 2 days with prior probenecid.
(4)   Other antibiotics used include amoxycillin, erythromycin, spiramycin, kanamycin, cephaloridine and cefuroxime.

Tetracycline, streptomycin, co-trimoxazole and choramphenicol are among drugs to be avoided in pregnancy. Treatment must take into account possible sensitivity to penicillin or ill-effects to the fetus. For the latter reference to the *Data Sheet Compendium* issued to all doctors in the United Kingdom is most useful. The safety of spectinomycin for use in pregnancy has not been established as yet, but an injection of this antibiotic appears to be effective treatment for penicillinase-producing gonococci found in recent years.

SYPHILIS
Syphilis is due to infection with the *Treponema pallidum* which is a spirochaete (a thin spiralled filamentous organism that dies very rapidly outside the host tissues). The disease can be acquired other

than venereally but only very rarely and by direct contact with the organism (such as by kissing an individual who has secondary syphilis and mouth lesions, or by a practitioner examining infected lesions carelessly. Soap and water kills the treponema).

The incubation period of the disease is from 10 to 90 days. The primary lesion or *chancre* appears usually as a painless indurated ulcer at the site of entry of the organism. This will heal and is generally not as obvious in the female (being usually sited on the labia) as in the male. *Secondary syphilis* is associated with a bloodstream infection and appears within a few months. Generally transient, the clinical features may include malaise, skin rashes, enlarged glands, anal condylomata and buccal ulcers. A latent phase will follow and it may be years before *tertiary syphilis* is manifest with its lesions or *gummata*. Skin, cardiovascular and central nervous systems are the areas mostly involved although some cases of spontaneous cure occur during the latent period.

Treated gonorrhoea can mask concomitant syphilis, but specialist departments will always follow up patients to ensure that treatment is adequate. Serological tests for syphilis include those that detect antibodies (reagin) in the blood of those with the disease. The Wassermann reaction (WR) and Kahn tests are now outdated as they are nonspecific and produce many false-positive results. The VDRL (venereal diseases research laboratory) slide test is used although this too detects reagin and produces false-positive results, as for example in patients with autoimmune diseases. Tests for treponemal antibodies include the TPHA (*Treponema pallidum* haemagglutination test) but other non-venereal treponemal infections rarely seen in the United Kingdom also react positively (such as yaws seen in the tropics, pinta in tropical America and bejel in the Middle East).

In syphilis the placenta is large, greasy and pale, and after its formation and in the mid-trimester of pregnancy the disease can cause abortion or intrauterine death. The treponema can also pass the placental barrier and cause congenital syphilis. Within a few weeks of birth the baby can show features of secondary syphilis and nasal discharge with 'snuffles' (loud nasal breathing). Later, gumma may collapse the bridge of the nose causing 'saddle nose', or there may be deformed teeth or radial scars around the mouth (rhagades); eyes, joints, central nervous system and ears may also be involved. Congenital syphilis is a rarity in the United Kingdom as treatment of the mother even late in pregnancy prevents the infection passing to the fetus. The routine serological tests to exclude the infection and performed at the initial prenatal examination is mandatory.

Treatment, usually with penicillin, is administered in various ways. An injection of 0.6 to 1.2 mega-units aqueous procaine penicillin daily for 10 days is widely used. Schedules using long-acting penicillins such as procaine penicillin in oil with aluminium monostearate (PAM) are also used, and these lessen the need for numerous injections and some involve one injection only of 2.4 or 4.8 mega-units for primary and secondary disease respectively. The venereologist is the best qualified to advise and arrange for follow-up tests. Erythromycin, on average 500 mg 6-hourly for 2 weeks, may be substituted if the patient is sensitive to penicillin.

TRICHOMONAS VAGINITIS
Trichomonas vaginitis (Figure 55) is caused by a pear-shaped flagellated protozoal organism which may be found in the urinary tract of men and women without causing symptoms. It may also be present in the vagina, but without a discharge. The protozoon may be identified under the microscope 'swimming' around most actively when a specimen of discharge is transferred directly to a slide containing a drop or two of saline (by the so-called 'hanging-drop' method).

Although infection is often contracted during coitus, this is not invariably so and indirect transmission by articles of clothing and towels is possible. The organism can also survive on a lavatory seat for some time. The discharge caused by trichomonas can usually be diag-

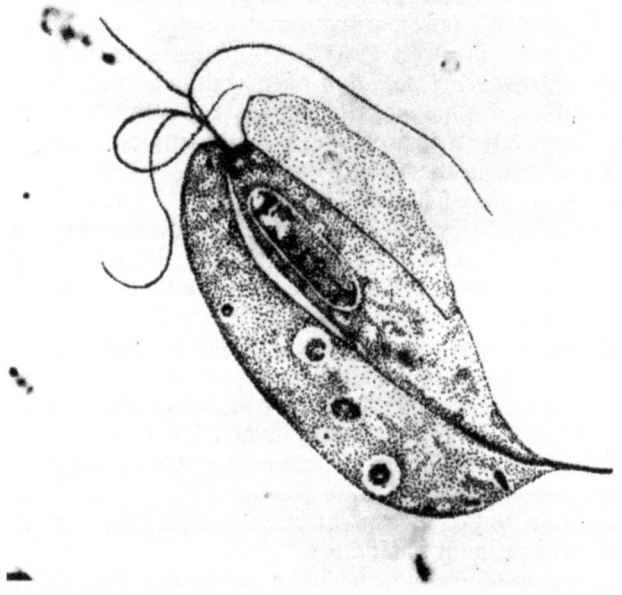

Figure 55   The protozoon *Trichomonas*

nosed by its three characteristics of being *watery, frothy* and *greenish* in colour. The possibility of a concomitant gonococcal infection should be borne in mind when trichomonas is found.

Treatment generally involves the use of a trichomonicide taken orally, and 200 mg tablets taken three times daily for 1 week is recommended. As the organism may possibly be introduced during coitus by a symptomless partner, a similar course to be taken concurrently by him may be prescribed. If such a course is prescribed, it is important to explain to the expectant mother the reasons for the step and name the causative organism as *Trichomonas vaginalis*, so that the patient and her husband are aware that gonorrhoea has not been diagnosed.

Although metronidazole is well tolerated and no adverse effects on the fetus have been found, therapy in the first 14 weeks of pregnancy is probably better deferred if possible.

CANDIDAL (MONILIAL) VAGINITIS (THRUSH)
The yeast-like fungus of *Candida albicans* (Figure 56) may be found as a saprophyte in the alimentary, upper respiratory and female genital tract, as well as on the skin of healthy people. Although many authorities consider candida is a normal and reasonably common inhabitant of a healthy vagina, this view is not universally accepted. If a vaginal swab reveals the presence of monilia and the patient complains of a vaginal discharge and/or pruritus, treatment should be instituted. The fact that candida prefers an acid vagina as found in pregnancy and flourishes in the presence of glycosuria has been discussed above (page 69).

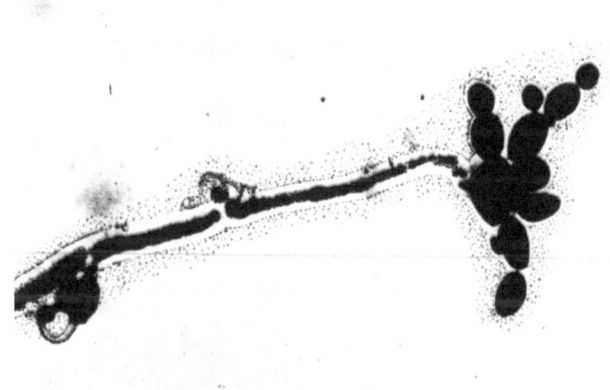

Figure 56   *Pseudomycelia* and spores of *Candida albicans*

Clinically the discharge may be recognized as thick creamy-white plaques which adhere to the epithelium and fill the rugae of the vaginal mucosa. The vagina in severe cases may contain masses of a cheese-like material which consists of pseudomycelia and spores of the fungus. The associated pruritus and vulvitis are often intolerable and result in insomnia and depression.

The forms of treatment were discussed above on page 69 and it may be necessary to repeat a course of treatment in pregnancy. I have seen many cases of persistent candidal vaginitis (also called thrush) in pregnancy whose symptoms have been controlled by treatment, but without completely eradicating the infection. Yet after vaginal delivery the patient was free of both symptoms and fungus! This is because during the second stage of labour the rugae of the vaginal mucosa unfold and the membrane becomes a smooth sheet (page 14), so the delivery of the infant and the escaping liquor carry away the fungus. (This is not to say, however, that the most effective treatment for candidal vaginitis is to have a baby!)

26

The rhesus factor and haemolytic disease

The Rh or rhesus factor, so-called because it is found in the blood of rhesus monkeys, is an antigen (that is, a substance capable of stimulating the formation of an antibody) found on the erythrocytes of 85−87% of Europeans who are described as Rh-positive. The antigen is not present in the red blood cells of the remaining 13−15% of the population who are Rh-negative. There is an ethnic variation in the percentages of population whose blood contains the Rh factor, and in many countries of the Far East Rh-negative blood is a rarity. The factor is inherited as a dominant Mendelian characteristic which means that an Rh-positive individual may be either homozygous when the factor is acquired from both parents, or heterozygous, from one parent only (see pages 34 to 36).

The Rh factor is a complex one and is made up of three pairs of

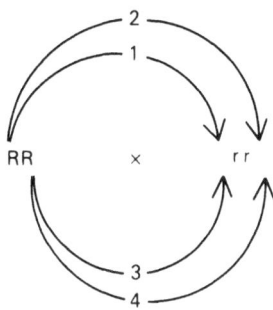

Homozygous Rh positive
father RR

Four possible combinations all
result in Rr (heterozygous Rh +)

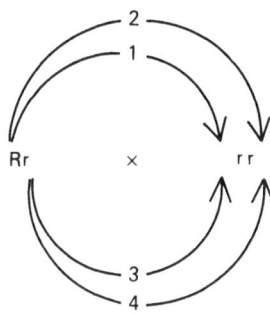

Heterozygous Rh positive
father Rr

Four possible combinations

1 = Rr ⎫
2 = Rr ⎬ i.e. 50% offspring
3 = rr ⎬ Rh negative
4 = rr ⎭

Figure 57 Inheritance of the Rhesus factor

229

allelomorphic genes known as Cc, Dd and Ee, the capital letter in each case (C, D and E) representing the dominant characteristic. For blood to be Rh-negative, C, D and E must all be absent, so the genotype which expresses status in relation to all three antigens is cde/cde. The commonest Rh antigen and one likely to cause isoimmunization is D.

A pregnant Rh-negative woman may have a Rh-positive fetus *in utero*, the Rh factor having been derived from the father. If the latter is homozygous Rh-positive every fetus must be Rh-positive, whereas if the father is heterozygous Rh positive 50% of the progeny will be Rh-negative. This may be seen in Figure 57 (the Rh factor has been simplified and represented by the letter R).

If during pregnancy, and especially at delivery, enough fetal cells with antigen D enter her bloodstream, the Rh-negative mother will react to them by producing antiD antibodies. The latter include the small immunoglobulins IgG (page 184) which can pass through the placenta to the fetus and cause haemolytic disease. A woman may have a baby *in utero* with blood of a different ABO group from her own, but if a similar transference of fetal blood cells took place the antibodies formed (macroimmunoglobulin IgM) are too big to traverse the placenta. Thus, only rarely does ABO incompatibility result in haemolytic disease. Fetal blood cells can enter the maternal bloodstream during labour, antepartum haemorrhage and abortion, during operations such as caesarean section or manual removal of the placenta, and during manoeuvres such as external cephalic version and amniocentesis. Some cells may escape spontaneously in the last weeks of pregnancy and enter the maternal bloodstream. As it takes many weeks for antibodies to develop the first child is very rarely affected, unless the mother has previously been sensitized by a transfusion of Rh-positive blood. However, once sensitized a woman will produce antibodies very rapidly if she receives even small quantities of D antigen on a future occasion, when subsequent Rh-positive babies are at risk.

Rh antibodies (*agglutinins*) which cross the placental barrier and enter the fetal bloodstream can cause fetal erythrocytes to agglutinate and rupture. This haemolysis liberates haemoglobin into the serum where it is converted into bilirubin.

Fetal haemolytic disease
Clinically, fetal haemolytic disease is manifest in three grades.

HAEMOLYTIC ANAEMIA OF THE NEWBORN
This is the least severe type and jaundice is not usually marked in the early days of life. Fetal haemoglobin which normally is about 18 g/100 ml (130%) should not fall below 14 g.

ICTERUS GRAVIS NEONATORUM

The anaemia is more severe and jaundice appears within 24 hours of birth and rapidly deepens. The baby's liver and spleen are enlarged (hepatomegaly and splenomegaly). If serum bilirubin is high (above 20 mg% as a rule) the child may develop *kernicterus*. In this condition the basal nuclei of the brain are jaundiced and the infant may die or suffer permanent brain damage.

HYDROPS FETALIS

Haemolysis and anaemia are so marked that intrauterine death occurs. In addition to hepatomegaly and splenomegaly the fetus is grossly oedematous, with effusions of fluid into abdomen, chest and pericardium. The condition is often associated with maternal hydramnios.

Reducing the adverse effects of Rh incompatibility isoimmunization

Measures which diminish the incidence or reduce the adverse effects of isoimmunization associated with Rh incompatibility include the following.

ROUTINE SCREENING

Blood tests taken at the initial prenatal visit of all women must include the determination of Rh status. If negative, the serum is examined for antibodies and efforts to establish the husband's grouping are made. Search for antibodies is repeated at 28 weeks and again at 34 weeks. If results are negative all is well, but at birth fetal (cord) blood is collected and examined for ABO group and Rh factor and haemoglobin is estimated. Coombs test uses an antigammaglobulin serum to detect antibodies. A direct positive result on fetal or cord blood indicates that the erythrocytes are coated with antibody, while an indirect positive test on maternal blood would mean that antibodies are present in her serum.

If antibodies are detected in the initial blood test prenatally, a titre is determined and where possible the husband's genotype is investigated. Maternal blood is re-examined at 24 weeks and monthly thereafter. A rising titre indicates that the fetus is probably affected and further investigation by amniocentesis should be performed. Mother and baby's interests are best served by further investigations and therapy as required being undertaken at centres specializing in this field. Spectrophotometric methods are employed to estimate the bilirubin content of the amniotic fluid.

TREATMENT

Treatment when a fetus is affected may be to administer an intraperitoneal transfusion to the fetus *in utero*, to induce labour before term or occasionally to perform caesarean section. Fetal blood is collected immediately on delivery and in addition to the tests mentioned above (ABO group, Rh status, haemoglobin estimation and Coombs test) the serum bilirubin is estimated. The baby may be given a simple blood transfusion to correct minor anaemia. If more severely affected (haemoglobin below 12 g/dl or bilirubin 14.5 mg/dl or more) the neonate is given an exchange transfusion via the umbilical vein. This must be administered within 12 hours of birth and Rh-negative blood of the same ABO group is used. Observations of the baby thereafter include regular serum bilirubin and haemoglobin estimations to ensure that there is no abnormal haemolysis.

PREVENTION

Sensitization of Rh-negative women who may have received Rh-positive fetal blood (cells with antigen D) can be prevented by intramuscular administration of RhD immunoglobulin (antiD gammaglobulin). The gammaglobulin reacts with the Rh-positive red cells neutralizing their antigenic effect. The injection should be given preferably within 24 hours and not later than 72 hours following possible sensitization (for example, following delivery or abortion). The dose of antiD gammaglobulin injected varies from 100 to 300 µg and the higher dose should be given if feto – maternal bleeding has been heavy (such as after caesarean section). The amount of feto–maternal blood transfer is determined by the *Kleihauer–Betke test*, a staining method whereby the number of fetal cells in the maternal blood can be counted. If the count is high, it should be repeated 72 hours later as occasionally more antiD gammaglobulin may be required. A dosage of only 50 µg appears to be adequate to prevent Rh isosensitization in conditions where feto–maternal blood transfer is probably slight, as for example in first-trimester vacuum abortion.

Trials in recent years suggest that immunoglobulin administered at the 28th week of pregnancy to all Rh-negative women with Rh-positive husbands is of value as a preventive measure. This prenatal administration may be worthwhile, but it is more important to ensure that *all* women at risk are given an appropriate injection immediately following any event that may cause sensitization to RhD antigen. Thus all cases of abortion and ectopic pregnancy in Rh-negative women with husbands whose blood type is either Rh-positive or unknown must be included.

27

The postnatal examination and family planning

The postnatal consultation and examination is usually best conducted 6 weeks after delivery. By this time involutionary processes as discussed in Chapter 22 should be either complete or nearly so, and in addition to the physical examination the consultation provides the opportunity:

(1) For the practitioner to advise the patient on any problems she may have concerning herself and/or her baby.
(2) To take cervical and vaginal smears.
(3) To make appropriate arrangements for

  (a) the investigation and treatment of conditions found prenatally and which were deferred because of the pregnancy;
  (b) long-term follow-up of conditions requiring this, such as hypertension, heart and renal diseases.

(4) To discuss family planning and procedures where required even though the topic had been discussed earlier in the puerperium.

Postnatal examination

The postnatal examination usually takes place in the general practitioner's surgery or in the hospital postnatal clinic. If the pregnancy ended unhappily, in that the baby was abnormal or failed to survive, both parents should be given a special appointment and be seen by a senior practitioner familiar with the circumstances. It may add to distress if the patient comes into contact with happy mothers and babies who were delivered at about the same time. Full discussion of the causes of an unfortunate outcome of pregnancy with advice about management and prognosis of a subsequent pregnancy is valuable.

After the patient has had the opportunity of discussing how she and her baby are progressing, the doctor should ask direct questions including:

Are you breast feeding? Are breasts and nipples completely comfortable? Is there any vaginal bleeding or discharge? If there is no bleeding, when did it (the lochia) stop? Are micturition and bowel action normal? Is there any pain or discomfort or are there any other problems?

The routine postnatal examination does not necessarily include a recording of blood pressure and urine analysis, provided these were completely normal throughout pregnancy. If, however, the patient suffered from pre-eclampsia or hypertension, or routine urine tests had shown any abnormality, these features must be checked. If not satisfactory the patient must remain under surveillance for further investigations and any necessary therapy. Furthermore, although it is important to ascertain the condition of breasts and nipples, there need be no examination if the patient is breastfeeding and without complaint. However, if there is any concern whatsoever, inspection and palpation of the breasts is essential.

Palpation of the abdomen should reveal no tumour and the uterus is not normally felt extending out of the pelvis. The tone of the abdominal wall musculature is noted and if flabby may be improved by exercises. Many mothers with young babies are unlikely to perform vigorous and time-consuming exercises such as leg, and head and shoulder-raising while recumbent, but may be prepared to contract the abdominal wall rhythmically while standing. This is an exercise to be encouraged and can be done concurrently while performing other household tasks.

The perineum and vulva are inspected and the labia gently separated as the patient is requested to bear down. This will demonstrate the integrity of the bladder, rectal and uterine supports. A minor degree of vaginal wall laxity usually improves with continued perineal exercises, and if necessary the condition can be reviewed after a few months. Pelvic examination includes inspection of the vagina and cervix, the taking of cervical and vaginal smears, and palpation of the perineal body, uterus and adnexal zones. There should be no pelvic tenderness.

POINTERS TO POSSIBLE ABNORMALITIES
Possible findings which may suggest abnormality include:

Vaginal discharge
Bacteriological examination of a high vaginal swab should be taken before deciding the nature of treatment, if any is necessary.

Vaginal granulations
A granulation may be found following imperfect healing of a laceration, especially in the posterior vaginal wall. This will often disappear after being touched *very lightly* with solid silver nitrate. If incorrect suturing has left the introitus too tight, the patient may be advised to stretch the pelvic floor digitally with two fingers in the vagina. The fingers should be anointed liberally with a lubricant jelly which may also be used initially when coitus is resumed.

Cervical erosion
An erosion is a red soft circumscribed and often granular area around the external os which is due to a replacement of the normal squamous epithelium by the columnar epithelium of the endocervical canal. The condition is common in pregnancy and is also a common finding at postnatal examination. It is generally hormonal in origin and may be associated with the oestrogen–progesterone balance. It is of interest to note that congenital cervical erosions are believed to be very common and associated with maternal oestrogens passed to the fetus. Outpatient treatment by electrocautery or by freezing with cryosurgery is unnecessary at the time of postnatal examination as the condition of the cervix is constantly varying. A review at a later date, however, is advised.

Pelvic tenderness
Tenderness may suggest infection and if present in the adnexal areas suggests pelvic cellulitis, thrombophlebitis or a haematoma. If other symptoms of infection are present antibiotic therapy may be necessary after bacteriological investigation of swabs.

Retrodisplacement of the uterus
A well-involuted mobile retrodisplaced uterus (see page 17) rarely causes symptoms such as backache and does not require active treatment. The patient may be advised occasionally to lie prone in bed and perform perineal exercises for another 6 weeks.

Continued bleeding
Although most mothers will have ceased to have a vaginal loss or discharge within 6 weeks of delivery, some complain of a slight blood loss which has persisted since the baby was born. If the uterus is fully involuted, the cervix closed and the lochial discharge diminishing progressively, there is probably no cause for concern. The clinical notes should be studied to verify that the placenta and membranes were delivered in their entirety, that blood loss during the third stage was not excessive, that lochia and involution initially were normal and that there was no pyrexia during the lying-in period. If all these features

are satisfactory no treatment is necessary but the patient should be reviewed within a week or two. If bleeding still continues, a pregnancy test is performed, and to ensure that no living chorionic tissue is present it must be negative. If any of the latter were retained *in utero* or anywhere in the body, there is a risk of chorioncarcinoma developing (see page 157).

The pregnancy test and treatment can be arranged at the first 6 weeks' examination if there is any concern. A course of oxytocic drugs such as oral ergometrine 0.5 mg three times daily for 3 days may be given prior to review. Evacuation of the uterus by dilatation and curettage is necessary if blood loss is heavy and there is a possibility of retained products of conception.

Atypical cells reported by the cytologist
Pregnancy provides an opportunity for cytological screening for all women and especially for those who have not had smears taken for some time. Carcinoma of the cervix is far more common in parous women and is related to sexual behaviour. The incidence is higher in those who commence coitus at an early age and those with many partners. In pregnancy with its changed hormonal status, epithelial activity is high, and some consider that examination of smears during pregnancy is desirable, but the test is often deferred until postnatal examination. If the cytologist reports the finding of atypical cells at this time, it is probably associated with the pregnancy but would indicate the need for repeat smears in 3 months.

Family planning
Although a family planning service involves all matters concerning contraception and subfertility, the latter is an unlikely topic for discussion at a postnatal examination! The increasing world population and the association of poor socioeconomic conditions and high parity have made contraception a subject of international importance, but not, however, for discussion here. As stated earlier, for those patients and their husbands who so wished, advice on family planning should have been given shortly after delivery, but the postnatal examination provides the opportunity for further discussion. The essentials of contraceptive practice merit consideration and the methods in common use are listed below with the main advantages and disadvantages.

CONTRACEPTIVE METHODS
The rhythm method or 'safe period'
This form of contraception relies upon the fact that after ovulation the mature ovum lives for approximately 1 day only, and although

living sperms have been found in the female body 7 days after deposition their effective life is probably much less. So there are only a few days each menstrual month during which pregnancy can occur. The time of ovulation is the most fertile period, and in view of the fact that sperms live longer than the ovum, coitus a day or two before ovulation is more likely to result in pregnancy than coitus occurring a day or two afterwards. The week preceding menstruation is the week during which pregnancy is least likely to occur.

It is usually stated that ovulation occurs 14 days before the next period, but this is not constant even when the menstrual cycle is regular, and only a minority of women have a very regular cycle. The basic body temperature recorded on waking rises after ovulation has occurred. The maintenance of a temperature chart for a limited period is of value when advising subfertile couples but it is not often kept for contraceptive purposes. It must be noted, however, that the temperature rise occurs not at the time of, but *after*, ovulation.

A strong motivation by those using the 'safe' period is necessary, and even then the failure rate is much higher than that associated with the sheath, diaphragm, IUD, or the Pill.

Coitus interruptus or 'withdrawal'
A widely used but not very effective form of contraception, as sperms may be present in fluid that escapes from the penis prior to ejaculation. The practice, however should not cause any physical or psychological trauma to couples using it.

Spermicidal pessaries, foams, creams or jellies
These are inserted into the vagina prior to coitus. The failure rate is high so the creams and jellies are of more value when used in conjunction with occlusive methods (see next paragraph).

Mechanical barriers
These prevent sperm and ovum meeting and include:

(1)   The condom or sheath, which if not defective, used correctly and throughout coitus, is an effective contraceptive device especially when used with spermicidal agents (see above).
(2)   The occlusive diaphragm or Dutch cap. A diaphragm is generally a thin latex rubber dome with a flexible circular rim, and the patient must be able to place it accurately in position. It is inserted into the vagina so that the posterior rim lies in the posterior fornix and the anterior rim is tucked away behind the symphysis pubis. The patient should be able to feel her cervix through the latex rubber to ensure that the device has been placed correctly to

occlude the upper vagina. A spermicidal cream or jelly is used as an adjunct to the cap which is inserted prior to intercourse and must not be removed for at least 6 hours.

In (2) above disadvantages of the need for expert fitting and the placing of the device in position before coitus are offset by the fact that the woman herself is controlling the contraceptive barrier and the sexual act is not interrupted as with (1) above. All women require re-fitting after a postnatal examination as the vaginal capacity may have changed.

Cervical caps which fit accurately over the cervix and are maintained in position by surface tension are rarely used.

Oral contraception − the Pill

The most efficient form of contraception when taken correctly is the combined pill which contains both oestrogen and progestogen. The great number of these products available makes for difficulty in choice, but a good principle to observe is to prescribe those that contain the smallest doses of hormones to be effective for the individual.

The oestrogen content of all combined pills has been progressively reduced so that today none contain more than $50\,\mu g$ of ethinyl oestradiol or mestranol. Oestrogen is responsible for many side-effects including thromboembolism, and the reduction from $100\,\mu g$ has diminished these effects without impairing contraceptive efficiency.

Combined pills are usually taken for 3 weeks in 4 and a course commences on the 5th day of a period. Progestogen-only pills (containing no oestrogen) commence on the 1st day of menstruation and medication is continuous. These so-called 'mini-pills' are not as effective as the combined pill, but they are of value when oestrogen administration is better avoided, such as during lactation and also in older women and diabetic patients.

The beneficial effects of the combined pill must be weighed against possible adverse effects. The latter receive wide publicity and may cause considerable anxiety, which may contraindicate the use of the hormones. One comprehensive textbook of gynaecology (Jeffcoate, 1975)* lists 24 side-effects of the pill and after commenting upon the 'formidable list' the author concludes that 'except for those women who are intolerant to oestrogen and those whose special circumstances contraindicate use of oestrogen−progestogen preparations, the modern contraceptive pill is virtually harmless'. Listed among oestrogenic effects are nausea, headache, breast tenderness, fluid retention and thromboembolism. Progestogen may cause depression, acne and

*Jeffcoate, N. (1975). *Principles of Gynaecology, 4th edition.* (London: Butterworths).

greasy scalp, leg cramps, increased appetite and scanty menstruation. Although most side-effects originally reported occur less commonly with low dosage pills, breakthrough bleeding may be more frequent, and if persistent for more than 3 months indicates the need for review.

Metabolic changes (probably oestrogenic in origin) seen in users of oral contraceptives include lowered carbohydrate tolerance, increase in plasma lipids and changes in liver function and folate metabolism. Other important complications include:

(1) *Hypertension*, which although usually slight, is occasionally significant. Blood pressure should be checked initially after 3 months of therapy, and then at least annually.

(2) *Thrombosis and embolism.* Oestrogenic effects include an increase in blood coagulability and thus an increased risk of developing deep vein thrombosis and thromboembolism. This risk increases with increasing age and weight and high tobacco consumption (cigarette smoking). The true incidence of fatal pulmonary emboli or cerebral thrombosis is difficult to determine, but the risk of death from all complications of any pregnancy is more than ten times greater than that associated with taking the contraceptive pill.

The risks of dangerous complications associated with the use of the combined pill must be considered in its true perspective, and the most important group of risks relates to the cardiovascular system. At present there appears to be no evidence that long-term usage might lead to cancer of the genital tract or breast, and smoking fifteen cigarettes or more a day would appear to be a greater hazard to life than taking the oral contraceptive. The small risk associated with the use of the latter is made very small indeed by identifying and excluding from therapy patients at special risk. These include women:

(1) over 40 years of age, or 35 if cigarette smokers;

(2) with a history of cardiovascular disease, deep vein thrombosis or thromboembolism, or hypertension;

(3) a history of breast cancer or certain other hormone-dependent conditions;

(4) with haemoglobinopathies, porphyria, or impaired liver function (see metabolic changes above);

(5) who are very adipose and with high blood lipids.

Other features to note are:

(1) Oestrogen-containing contraceptive pills should not be taken by a patient who is to undergo major surgery within 6 weeks, or by

patients who are not ambulant for any reason. Both these conditions may predispose to deep vein thrombosis.

(2) Hormonal contraception must not be prescribed if there is a possibility of a pregnancy.

(3) Other contraceptive methods should also be used in the first 2 weeks of medication.

(4) Secondary amenorrhoea which may sometimes occur may lead to considerable concern. The patient should be examined and if there is no uterine enlargement and a pregnancy test is negative she can be reassured if taking the combined pill regularly.

Post-pill amenorrhoea often takes up to a year to correct spontaneously but thereafter may require investigation and therapy.

(5) Psychological disturbances, depression or loss of libido are occasionally reported as associated with pill usage. There are often, however, underlying causes for these symptoms which are not directly attributable to the hormone being taken.

The intrauterine device (IUD)

The unfortunate habit of using initials to represent words, even in conversation, is so widespread that it is now accepted practice. It remains, however, a practice to be deprecated, and especially where the initials IUD are used, as to every doctor and midwife in the United Kingdom a generation ago, the letters IUD meant intrauterine death. However, the author's attempt to have the letter C inserted universally so that the device became an IUCD was too localized to be effective!

The intrauterine contraceptive device comes in many shapes and forms and has the advantage that if retained in the uterine cavity no further measures need to be taken to prevent pregnancy. Its disadvantages include possible resultant menorrhagia and abdominal cramps, although the latter will probably disappear after a few menstrual cycles. Devices should be inserted by an experienced practitioner using antiseptic and aseptic techniques to avoid the risk of introducing infection. The rare risk of perforating the uterus will be minimized if force is never used to insert a uterine sound or dilator (to measure the length of cervical and uterine cavity), or when inserting the device. Nearly 10% of appliances may be expelled spontaneously, and the patient should be advised to inspect vulval pads especially in the early months to ensure that this has not occurred.

IUDs are made mostly of inert plastic polyethylene and are straightened as they are placed into the introducer immediately prior to use, but revert to their manufactured shape inside the uterus.

Most devices which incorporate copper wire around one of the 'limbs' (the Copper 7, for example) should be renewed every 2 years, but others now being used (such as Copper T 200 and Copper T 380) are reputedly more efficient, have a lower expulsion rate and may be left *in utero* for much longer. It is claimed that the copper increases contraceptive efficiency. Other non-metallic-containing devices may be left *in situ* for many years and some authorities consider that the IUD may remain for as long as the patient wishes if it is causing no untoward symptoms.

The mode of action of the IUD is uncertain. More than 50 years ago the Gräfenberg ring of silver wire was first inserted *in utero* and achieved some popularity in European countries but not in the United Kingdom. It was thought to act by causing endometritis, although the infection may have been introduced at its insertion. IUDs do, in fact, provoke an inflammatory response which is not due to bacterial invasion, and this response produces a high concentration of leukoyctes and macrophages which have a phagocytic action on sperms. Furthermore the level of prostaglandins in the endometrium is increased with an associated increase in myometrial contraction which may prevent implantation.

Some IUDs contain a reservoir of progesterone which is reported to be released at a controlled rate and these require annual replacement. They are not recommended for use at this stage in their development.

STERILIZATION

Full discussion regarding sterilization in the puerperium should take place between doctor, patient and her husband weeks or months before delivery and not during labour or in the immediate postpartum days. Although methods of operation and appliances for temporary female sterilization are available, it is preferable to regard the procedure as irreversible, and the patient should be so informed even though surgery to establish fertility after bilateral tubal occlusion may succeed. The small risks of the procedure and the fact that not quite 100% success rate can be guaranteed with tubal sterilization operations must be pointed out, but this must not be overstressed in case the patient loses confidence in the procedure.

The percentage of women who request reversal of sterilization is higher when the procedure is performed in the puerperium, and in younger patients of low parity. A post-tubal sterilization syndrome has been described and many experts believe that there is a greater incidence of pelvic pain and irregular bleeding in women who have been subject to operation. However, others consider that the procedure itself is not the agent responsible for the symptoms. Furthermore, if a woman aged 40 or more has these gynaecological symptoms and there are grounds for sterilization, the possibility that a hysterectomy may be more beneficial should be considered. These factors, the reasons for requesting sterilization and other means of contraception (including vasectomy for the husband) are all considered when the parents are being counselled. It is also advisable to consult the patient's general practitioner who will know more about the patient and her social conditions than the hospital specialist.

Techniques for female sterilization
These include

(1) *Laparoscopy*, in which:

   (a) the tubes are occluded by electrocoagulation in two zones on each side, and the intervening tubal area may or may not be divided, or
   (b) a ring or band, or a clip is applied to the tubes. This obviates the risk of heat damage by electricity to other organs and is more readily reversible.

(2) *Laparotomy*. A so-called minilaparotomy via a small transverse suprapubic incision is the method preferred by many for postpartum sterilization. The fallopian tubes may be ligated and cut, excised or occluded with rings or clips. Reversible sterilization can sometimes be achieved by burying the fimbriated ends of the tubes between the layers of the broad ligaments. The minilaparotomy performed a few days after delivery should not increase the patient's length of stay in hospital. The fallopian tubes in the immediate postpartum period tend to be vascular and oedematous, so the risk of haemorrhage is increased if laparoscopy electrocautery is used. Also an increased failure rate is reported when clips or rings are used for tubal occlusion. The tubal condition postpartum makes a vaginal approach via the posterior fornix (*posterior colpotomy*) less satisfactory even in the hands of those experienced in this method.

If delivery is by caesarean section tubal sterilization can be performed simultaneously when indicated, but the decision for this should have been made long before the operation. Whereas sterilization may be offered to all women having a third caesarean section, it is now common practice for the obstetrician to agree to the procedure if requested when the patient is over 30 years of age. Caesarean section, however, is not performed solely because sterilization is indicated.

The efficiency of the various methods of contraception is usually expressed numerically by quoting failure rates per 100 woman-years. The figure would thus indicate the number of pregnancies that may be seen annually in 100 couples using a particular method. Reported rates show a very wide variation, and apart from sterilization procedures, this variation can be explained by differences in motivation. The figures in Table 2 are thus approximate and compiled from several sources.

Table 2   Failure rate per 100 woman-years

Sterilization	0.2−0.3	(for laparoscopy cautery or rings; rate is higher when clips are used and lower when mini-laparotomy performed as described)
Combined pill	0.1−0.6	
Progestogen-only pill	2−3	
IUD	2−3	(if retained in utero)
Sheath or diaphragm	2−20	(lower figure when properly used)

28

The breasts

Anatomy of the breasts

The female breasts which at birth consist almost wholly of a group of straight tubules of ectodermal origin, begin to develop at puberty when the ducts commence to branch, fat is deposited subcutaneously and fibrous tissue increases in amount. After puberty, ovarian oestrogens cause the ductal system to elongate and branch, and buds form in the distal part of the branches. These buds or clusters of cells are the potential breast alveoli and the formation and further development is induced by progesterone. Other hormones, too, are involved in breast development including thyroid and adrenal secretions, pituitary growth hormone (somatotrophin) and prolactin.

The mature breast extends from the second to the sixth rib vertically, and from the side of the sternum to the axillary line. A projection of breast tissue, the *axillary tail*, passes from the superolateral zone to the axilla. Loose areolar tissue and a layer of deep fascia separates the breast from the muscles of the anterior chest wall, mainly the pectoralis major. The gland tissue is arranged in 15 to 20 lobes which are separated from each other by fibrous and adipose tissue. The lobules comprising each lobe consist of clusters of alveoli which open into small ducts. The *alveolar ducts* unite to form the *lactiferous ducts*. The latter, one of which comes from each lobe, converge to the nipple, but before reaching it each forms a dilatation or *ampulla* in which milk can be stored. The nipple contains unstriped muscle fibres and 15 to 20 minute orifices on the tip which are the openings of the lactiferous ducts. The circular area of skin around the base of the nipple, the *areola*, becomes pigmented in pregnancy while its sebaceous glands enlarge and are known as *Montgomery's tubercles* (Figure 58).

Secretory activity in the alveoli is seen normally only in association with pregnancy during which increasing amounts of oestrogen and progesterone from the placenta cause marked increase in ductal development associated with increased vascularity and amounts of adipose

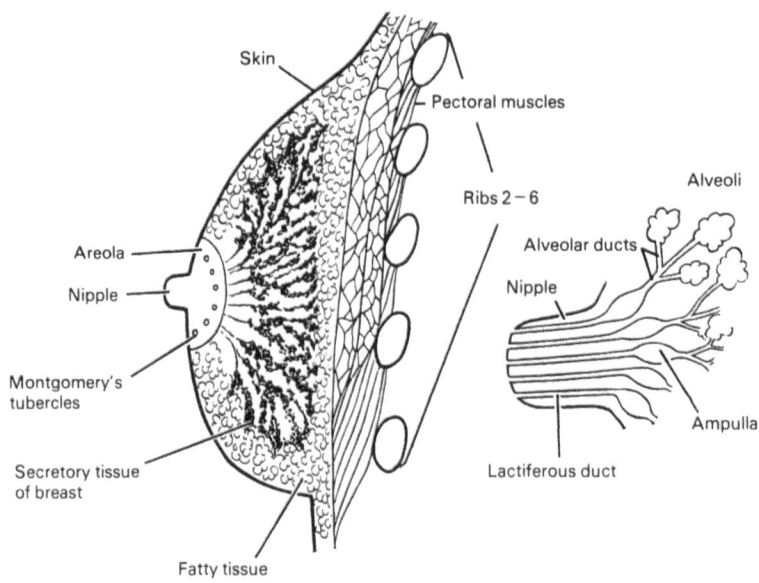

Figure 58 The breast

tissue. *Colostrum*, a turbid fatty secretion, is found in the second half of pregnancy and for the first few days postpartum, and true milk does not appear until about the 3rd day following parturition. Lactation is initiated by the anterior pituitary hormone *prolactin*, the release of which is dependent on the levels of oestrogen and progesterone. A high level inhibits the release of prolactin by acting through the hypothalamus and stimulating the secretion of prolactin inhibiting factor (PIF). Following delivery a rapid fall of the blood levels of oestrogen and progesterone occurs, and this triggers off the production of prolactin.

Suckling stimulates the numerous nerves in and around the nipple, and by a reflex action oxytocin is released from the hypothalamus and neurohypophysis (posterior pituitary). This hormone stimulates the involuntary muscular elements (*myoepithethial cells*) around the alveoli and ducts, thus causing the flow of milk. The regular stimulation of the nipple by suckling and emptying the breasts is a most important factor in maintaining milk flow. The oxytocin produced also stimulates uterine contractions, promotes lochial flow and is the cause of some women experiencing 'after-pains' while breastfeeding.

Breastfeeding the baby is to be preferred because apart from supplying the most suitably balanced and sterile nutrition at the correct temperature, it provides protection against certain infections. Studies in recent years have shown that breast milk contains immuno-globulins, lactoferrin and enzymes that can protect against bacterial invasion (*lysozyme*), and that it is also a prophylactic against food allergy in infancy. Breastfeeding is an important factor in establishing a close relationship between mother and baby (*bonding*). The stimulation of prolactin secretion by regular breastfeeding also has a limited contraceptive effect (but see Chapter 27) and even though reports state that half the women in some developing countries become pregnant while breastfeeding, the latter does play a part in child spacing.

Some patients with inadequate breasts or anchored inverted nipples may wish to make excessive efforts to satisfy their desire to feed the baby, while a small percentage find even the thought of breastfeeding repugnant. Expectant mothers may be persuaded to breastfeed by reasoning, but they must not be coerced. The patient's peace of mind is important.

Prenatal care of the breasts in preparation for breastfeeding varies. Some authorities recommend regular massage of the tissues towards the nipple which is then gently pulled out; the procedure is repeated several times daily. Such a recommendation is not made in my units. Breasts are examined routinely initially and again at about 32 weeks, and more frequently if necessary. If all is normal no special recommendations are made except:

(1)   to wash the nipples daily with soap and water which is usually adequate to avoid crusting, and
(2)   to wear a comfortable brassière that supports the weight of the breasts without compression.

Inverted nipples that are not anchored may be improved by the wearing of 'shells', or the patient can be instructed gently to ease the nipple out digitally and apply lanolin or baby oil.

Soon after delivery the mother is given her baby to suckle, and this is done at regular intervals slowly increasing the time at the breast to 10 minutes each side on the 3rd day. Initially only small amounts of colostrum are obtained. When lactation is established feeding on demand is the general practice. Successful breastfeeding requires not only an adequate supply of milk to a normal infant from normal breasts and nipples, but also a mother who is well, not anaemic and psychologically well adjusted. The mother should be comfortably settled in bed or chair, supervised initially by a skilled attendant and the general atmosphere in the room or ward should be one of contented tranquillity.

Breast engorgement

Breast engorgement is not uncommon and occurs on the 3rd or 4th day postpartum as lactation is being established. The breasts become generally tense, hot and tender as a result of venous and lymphatic engorgement. Distended veins coursing superficially across the breasts are often visible. The tenseness obstructs the lactiferous ducts and the milk cannot flow. A low-grade pyrexia commonly accompanies the condition.

Treatment aims at keeping the patient as comfortable as possible as the condition usually settles quickly when the milk begins to flow and the baby can suckle and empty the breast. A supporting but not too tight brassière and simple analgesics such as soluble aspirin will help. Local applications, either hot packs or icebags, are applied by experienced midwives with seemingly equal effect! A gentle but effective breast pump to drain off some milk before the baby feeds is often useful. Oxytocin given either by injection, nasal spray or buccal pitocin is used. Stilboestrol in 5 mg doses is still used with effect, but this hormone is better avoided completely.

Engorgement of the breasts may occasionally be associated with capillary bleeding which can colour the milk. Provided the bleeding is very slight and settles within a few days, breastfeeding is permissible although it is desirable to have bacteriological examination of a swab and cytological examination of a specimen of the discharge. It is important to exclude the possibility of a duct papilloma as the causative factor. If bleeding is persistent or heavy it may be necessary to inhibit lactation.

Bloodstained discharge from the nipple during pregnancy also occurs for similar reasons. The breasts should always be examined to exclude pathology.

Cracked nipples and mastitis

Small fissures in the epithelium covering the nipples are often due to faulty technique in breastfeeding, but sometimes they are associated with abnormalities in the nipple itself or overaggressive suckling. Cracked nipples are painful and form the most common portal of entry for bacteria which initiate acute mastitis and breast abscess. If, therefore, the patient complains of any pain when the baby feeds, careful examination of the nipple and areola, with a lens if necessary, is essential. Cracked nipples usually heal within a day or two if rested and local applications such as tincture benzoin may be used but these are of secondary importance to resting the nipple. Nipple shields which afford protection during suckling are also of value.

Infection of the breast tissue, *acute mastitis*, is often due to

Staphylococcus aureus derived from the baby (see page 207), but many other organisms may be involved. Mastitis develops later in the puerperium, often between the 2nd and 4th week and is associated with pain and tenderness over an inflamed, hot, indurated breast. Pyrexia may be high and the patient toxic with severe malaise. Rigors are possible.

Avoidance of acute mastitis by meticulous nipple care and early treatment of cracks is undoubtedly better than having to deal with the developed condition, but the latter, however, can occasionally arise from a bloodstream infection. Treatment of mastitis after bacteriological examination of the milk includes rest, analgesics and broad-spectrum antibiotic therapy. Breasts must be emptied regularly, and if the milk is sterile and suckling not too painful the baby may continue to breastfeed. If, however, the milk is infected or breasts too painful, a pump is used.

A breast abscess presents as a fluctuating tender area with induration as the purulent collection becomes walled off by fibrosis. Antibiotic therapy is often given but is usually unhelpful in eliminating a localized abscess. Treatment entails adequate incision and draining performed under general anaesthesia. It may take many days for a suspected abscess to become localized and 'ripe' for incision, especially when it is deepseated in origin. A breast abscess rarely endangers life, but it can make a mother feel wretched.

Inhibition of lactation

It is usually easier to inhibit lactation than it is to suppress it when established. Oestrogens used in the past for this purpose should be avoided as they increase the risk of thrombosis. The strict avoidance of any form of breast stimulation after delivery coupled with the wearing of a firm supporting brassière are usually the only measures required to inhibit lactation. If discomfort is experienced at about the 3rd day, soluble aspirin may be administered. Fluid intake need not necessarily be severely restricted, and purgation and the binding of breasts are totally unnecessary. If medication other than simple analgesics is required, bromocriptine 2.5 mg tablets taken twice daily with food for 14 days is the drug of choice. Bromocriptine inhibits secretion of prolactin by the pituitary, and the course stated is used for both inhibition and suppression of lactation.

The axillary tail may sometimes contain active secretory alveoli and thus swells when lactation is established on about the 3rd day postpartum. The soft axillary swelling is not unduly tender and no special treatment is indicated. Functioning ectopic breast tissue elsewhere in the body may be present, but it is rare.

Index

os pubis   2
  incompetent   151
ovaries
  components   20, 21
  cortex   20
  cyclical changes   24−7
  medulla   21
  position   20
ovulation   24−6
  animals   32
  hormones and   26
ovum   25
  blighted   150
oxytocin   74, 84, 97, 157, 177, 178, 247
  and induction   196
  infusion   180

pain relief in labour   98−101
papaveretum   98
para-aminosalicylic acid   221
paracervical block   101
paraldehyde   142
paraurethral ducts   13
parietal bone   8, 9
  eminence   8, 9
partogram and labour monitoring   96, 97
Pawlik grip   55
pelvic cavity   4, 5, 168
pelvic inlet   3
  boundaries   4
  and fetal position   53
pelvic outlet   3, 5, 168
  assessment   6, 8
  contracted   169
pelvic planes   5
  erect   5
pelvic viscera view   15
pelvimetry, internal   5, 6
  external   6
  radiological   6, 8
  X-ray   172, 173
pelvis
  anatomy   1−5, 167−9
  android   168
  anthropoid   169
  bones   1−3

clinical examination   4−8
contracted   167−9
  diagnosis   169−73
diagonal conjugate diameter   6
disproportion   167−73, 178, 195
  management   173
false and true   3
gynaecoid   168, 170
measurements   171
platypelloid   168, 169
stretching   1
types   167−9
penicillin   216, 224
  procaine   225, 226
pentazocine   99
perimetrium   17
perineum tears   202, 203
pethidine   98, 144
placenta
  adhesions   78
  barrier   184
  circumvallate   186, 187
  cord traction   80, 81
  delivery   72, 76, 80, 81
  development control   34
  formation   31−3
  functions   183, 184
  hourglass contraction ring   78, 79
  manual removal   82, 83
  monitoring of efficiency   190, 191, 220
  praevia   111, 158, 162−6
    delivery   165
    examination   164, 165
    mortality   165, 166
    symptoms   163, 164
    treatment   165
    types   163
    vaginal examination   165
  and pre-eclampsia   133
  retained
    causes   78
    treatment   81−4
placental insufficiency   183
polycystic ovarian disease   38, 63
postnatal examination   233−6
postpartum haematoma   84
postpartum haemorrhage

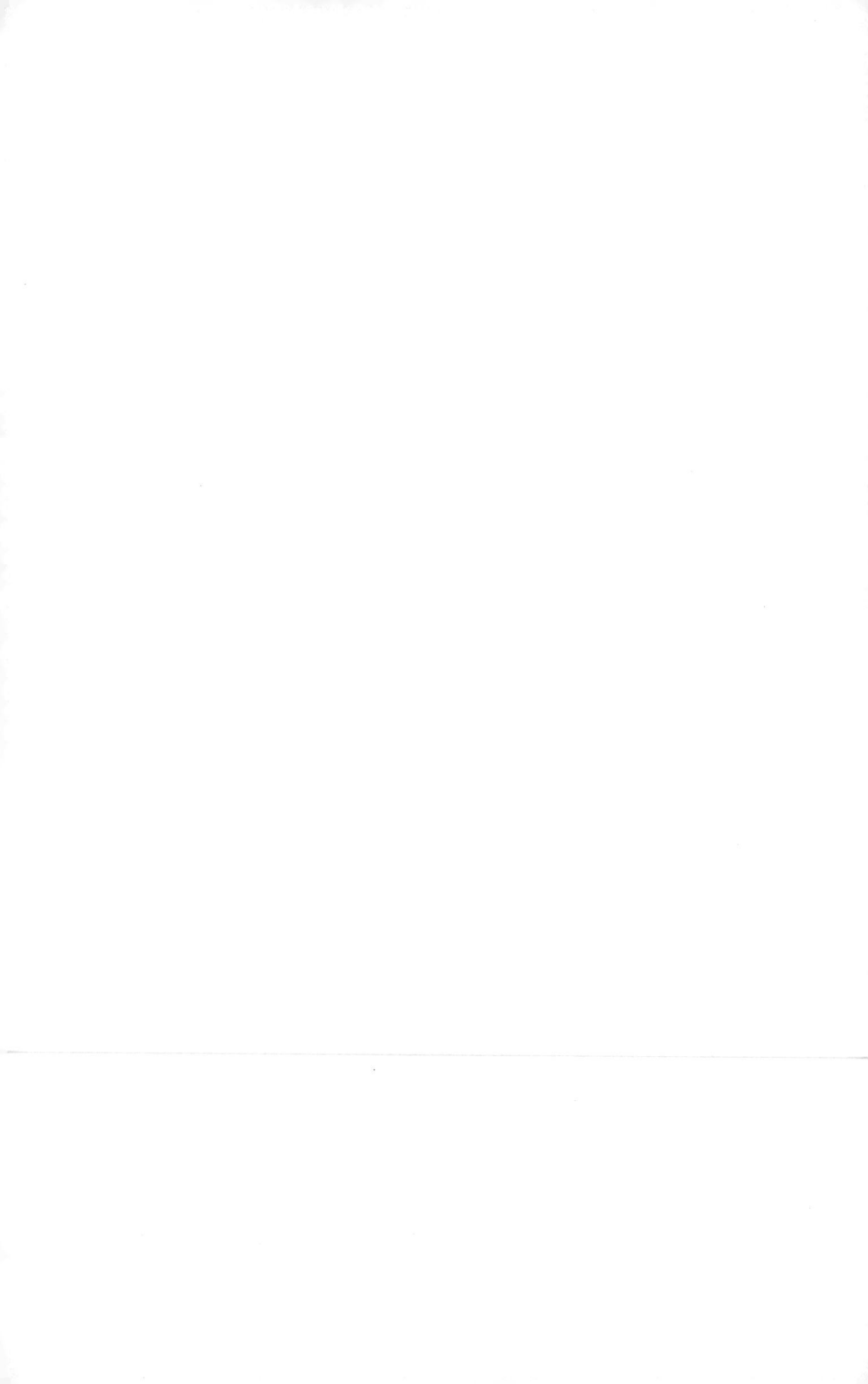